IT'S NOT OVER YET!

When a woman reaches a certain age, she comes to a crossroads: Will she try to stay young as a:

- "Daisy Dukes and Ugg Boots lady," OR will she resign herself to be a frumpy
- "Sweatpants and Baseball Cap lady" OR continue to ROCK IT as a still head-turning
- "I Love My **Beauty Power!** lady"?

In **"It's Not Over Yet!,"** **Sally Van Swearingen** reveals HOW TO reclaim YOUR beauty edge as you move into your second half of life; rediscovering the joys of getting gorgeous in an age-adapted but sexy and playful way.

Sally shares her funny and insightful personal revelations, her own "get-a-clue" journey that brought her back from "Post-40 Invisible Mom" to "50s and Fabulous Hottie." She also shares insider beauty secrets and wisdom she has gained by making over 5,000 women even more beautiful.

"If I can do it, YOU can do it!"
says beauty guru Sally Van Swearingen.

IT'S NOT OVER YET!

To Chanty,

Sally
VAN SWEARINGEN

a great a
artist and a
beautiful lady!
Here's to your
Beauty Power!
- Sally

IT'S NOT OVER YET!

Reclaiming Your REAL Beauty Power in Your 40s, 50s and Beyond

Sally Van Swearingen

IT'S NOT OVER YET!

IT'S NOT OVER YET! Reclaiming Your Real Beauty
Power
in Your 40s, 50s and Beyond

Published by

Beauty Power Ink

Third Printing

Copyright © 2014 by Sally Van Swearingen

ISBN: 978-0-9903047-6-0

Printed in the United States of America

NOTHING MAKES A

Woman

MORE *Beautiful*

THAN THE BELIEF

THAT SHE IS

Beautiful

IT'S NOT OVER YET!

My heartfelt thanks to the smart, focused, life changing "Sally wranglers:" Matt Randall, for putting this project, (and me!) at the top of his list, and Judith Cassis, who insisted that I must write this book for all women.

You are my role models.

And thanks to all my gorgeous **Beauty Power** clients who have trusted me with their faces and hair.

I love my job.

"Associate yourself with people of good quality, for it is better to be alone than in bad company."

—Booker T. Washington

Sally VAN SWEARINGEN

IT'S NOT OVER YET!

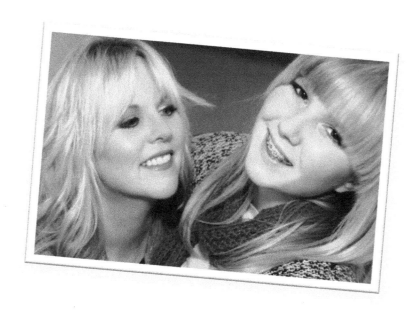

To my mama, Eleanore, and to my loving family,
whose strength is a force to be reckoned with.

And to my beautiful and smart daughter,
Brigitte Rose,
whose presence has always given my life
direction.

It's Not Over Yet!

Forward

"Sally Van Swearingen is my go-to person for beauty. Why? Because she gets it!

She not only works in the beauty and entertainment industry, she lives it every day.

After reading "It's Not Over Yet!"... Guess what? It never WILL be!

A breath of fresh air to all of us who have been told we are past our prime.

Of course, in Hollywood, that means anyone over 30!

This book is a must read for any woman of "a certain age."

I give "It's Not Over Yet!" an A+! No wonder she's on the A List!"

—Bella Shaw, Former CNN anchor, ageless! (55+)

On my way now to pick up the faux lashes Sally recommends, but wait, there's more!

I have a whole list of things I want to try!

"When I met Sally I was told she had just turned 50...
I looked at her and thought, whatever she is selling, I
want it."
—Arlyne Szerman, 65

"Women 35+ rejoice! We've got Sally!"
—Cynthia Moller, 49

"It was my 40th birthday. I had to look great, but had
run out of ideas. Sally showed me a few "tricks of the
trade" to update my look, and I got a little too much
attention on my birthday!"
—Alice Mecom, 44

"Creating alchemy. That's Sally, mixing beauty with
heart."
—Christine Gron, 63

"As a makeup artist, Sally is modern, intuitive and
extraordinarily talented. My daughters are grown, and
now it's 'me' time. Sally gets it."
—Lisa Howard, 43

"Being a professional speaker, my image is often
projected onto a huge screen. Sally's quick beauty
tricks take me from zero to **Beauty Power.** I feel so
confident because I know I'm looking good!"
—Judith Cassis, 54

IT'S NOT OVER YET!

Table of Contents

IT'S NOT OVER YET!

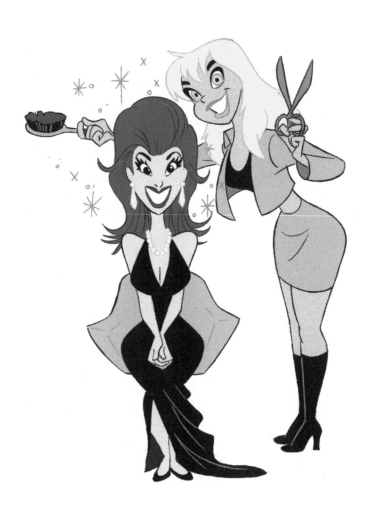

Introduction

I believe one of the reasons I have been put on this earth is to help ladies love themselves more, beauty challenges and all.

In my salon, The A LIST Hair and Makeup Studio, my clients are my personal Barbie dolls! I feel actual JOY showing ladies how to reclaim their **Beauty Power.**

Previous to my current passion as a salon owner and freelance makeup artist, I created a bridal makeup studio that turned out thousands of gorgeous Southern California brides!

I'm qualified to write this book because:

- I have personally made up over 5,000 faces.

- I have worked behind the camera for over twenty years on photo shoots, commercials, infomercials and videos.

- I have been on camera numerous times and have assisted others with creating a flawless image.

- I have traveled the U.S. and Canada as a platform makeup educator.

I would say that my life's work has been to bring out the total beauty in every woman I have worked with. I truly love my job and have never tired of it. I also know a thing or two about growing up a pretty, vivacious blonde and being content with it, taking it for granted, then seeing my beauty power slipping away after childbirth, weight gain and aging. People treated me differently. In my business, doors didn't open as easily as before. I had to PUSH them open!

I had almost accepted that part of my life was over.

In our youth, we fail to realize how much POWER our good looks play into our success in relationships, business and life in general. When we find things don't come to us as easily as in our teens through 30s, we unfortunately face the music that we may have lost our **Beauty Power**.

Some of us just give up and accept it. Others realize that it is NOT TOO LATE to look and feel beauty-licious!

The following is my personal story about how I reclaimed my **Beauty Power** and how you can too!

You may not always agree with my views, and even if you don't, enjoy. Listen to my story. It may or may not be similar to your own.

My desire is that you walk away from reading this book inspired and geared up to reclaim your own **Beauty Power.**

What do I want to accomplish with this journey? My greatest wish is that you will experience a mind shift, a move toward self-love and empowerment, AND be inspired to take action every day to bring out your inner and outer hottie, no matter what your age.

After reading It's Not Over Yet!, you will be a step closer to embracing the fact that we each have our own unique "It factor." The thing about you that shines when you enter a room. You will begin to reveal this special gift only YOU have.

Ladies, this isn't a sweet little beauty book you relax with and read on a Sunday afternoon. My goal is to inspire you to work on your **Beauty Power** starting right now.

Let's do this thing!

Why did you buy this book? What are you looking to accomplish?

_____

_____

_____

_____

My Philosophy on Personal Beauty Power:

What is it?

What do I know now after spending 25 years as a beauty professional?

What makes a woman of any age attractive and appealing is that uniqueness we put out there. I'm going to give you examples of **Beauty Power** winners!

Who has Beauty Power?

I have a friend who is a working dancer at the age of 40. She's fit, small-breasted and slender, such a beauty in a strong way. Her sculpted cheekbones and well-toned arms are things to covet. She could be wearing simple dance pants and a T-shirt and she looks absolutely beautiful. She comes into the dressing room at the dance studio where we take class. We often talk as she puts on her makeup. I have made her up for on-camera, yet it's without makeup that I find her the most stunning. She has **Beauty Power**..

A vivacious, coppery redheaded client of mine is curvalicious, tall and broad, with full breasts and hips. Her look reminds me of a line from a 1990s club dance song that says "red beans and rice didn't miss her." (Remember it? We all grooved to it!) She always inspires me with some cute, trendy outfit, proudly playing up her voluptuousness. Her eclectic, frisky fashion sense makes me want to run out of my salon and beeline to the mall with her, right now! She is powerful, sexy and certainly

"Curvalicious" when she enters a room. She has **Beauty Power.**

My beautiful sister, Robin, is fit at 58. Her passions are baking, cooking and clothes. Because she loves to wear great clothes and eat good food, she works out and takes care of herself. Sis puts out a conservative style, classy and harmonious. She believes a woman should wear clothes that showcase her individual style while enhancing her body shape. When Robin walks into a room, the first thing you notice is that she is put together. She takes the time to design her look before going out the door, even if it is simply jeans, boots and a sweater for movie night. She is a clever connoisseur of fashion and manages to put great looks together within her budget. For example, she showed up recently wearing a vintage motorcycle jacket. As I began to drool, she happily reported that she discovered it at the local consignment store! This woman knows how to shop. She has **Beauty Power.**

Each one of these ladies is admired, and often complimented by others, for her personal style.

We must develop OUR personal style and move to our own unique rhythm, as we discover the next chapter and what is waiting for us right around the bend.

My Personal Style

The personal style I'm redesigning at this time of my life is not too far from what I put out in my 30s, yet age-appropriate. I call it Classic Edgy. A little rock and roll, with classic lines, fitted, closer to the body, lots of basic black with some cheetah print or fun jewelry, but I also remember that I'm in my 50s; certain looks don't work for me anymore.

That would include skirts that are too short. Even if you have good legs (I do), too far above the knee says "trashy." Blouses cut too low say "advertising for attention." Keep boob-baring blouses for your private date nights.

However, this doesn't mean I'm going to totally cover myself up because I'm past a certain age, and neither should YOU!

A few years ago Judith Cassis, my book coach and good friend, observed some fashion behavior in me that she just didn't get. She noticed that when I walked onto a stage or in front of a camera, I dressed conservatively... business suit or jacketed black dress, fully covered. However, in everyday life she would find me in curvy, fitted dresses and high heels, or black jeans and boots, topped with a leather jacket. She wanted to know WHY I completely changed my look to be "beauty executive" on stage.

I explained that I wanted to be seen as an expert beauty guru. Judith pondered that for a few minutes, then shared with me- that for people to truly "get" you, you need to be your authentic self always, no matter what your platform. She offered, "How will you get the message across, about being attractive and appealing at any age, while you are changing into someone you are not?" That was a HUGE epiphany for me. Thanks, Judith! That observation may well have been the beginning of this book. It's Not Over Yet!

IT'S NOT OVER YET!

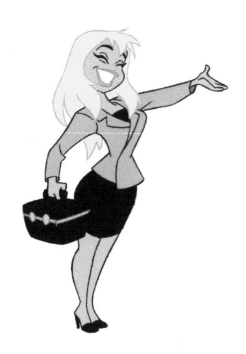

CHAPTER 1

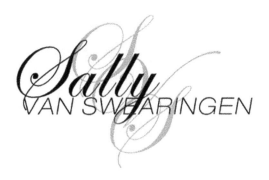

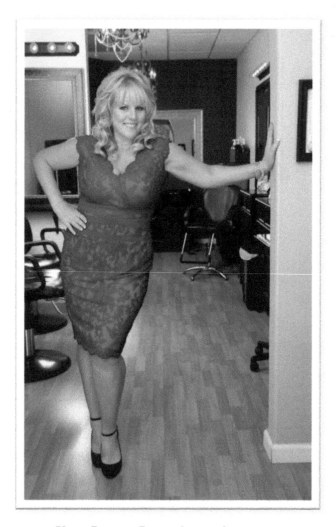

Your Beauty Power begins here

Personal Development from my Own Life Lessons: Reclaiming Your Beauty Power

Life Lesson #1: Get a Clue

Looking younger than my actual age has proven to be a benefit in my industries: beauty and entertainment.

When not working as a makeup artist on set or in my Santa Clarita studio, I am occasionally guilty of looking like a tired, stressed-out mom. Sadly, I do see this look on other ladies too; no makeup, baggy clothes, racing around town, trying to get too many errands done in a day. Most days I take the time to look the part. My point is that I am very clear about how people judge, and how we are viewed. Are YOU clear?

It became CRYSTAL clear to me one day in the bank, back in 2001, when my daughter Brigitte was just a baby. I was sporting a typical new mom getup: baggy dress, hair in a clip, no makeup and, yes, the trick many of us use to escape the glare of inspections, dark sunglasses. I struck up a conversation with a mature (mature here means older than me ☺), attractive woman in line beside me, and we conversed about our lives. "What do you do?" she inquired. My answer came out confidently, accompanied by a proud smile. "I'm in the BEAUTY business. A makeup artist. Mostly commercials and brides. Actually, I am now creating a makeup kit for brides." She studied me hard and quick. "REALLY?" her eyes bearing a doubtful and surprised look. She obviously wouldn't have guessed that one.

BING! That life-changing phenomenon called the "aha" moment. As I carried my baby girl out of the bank, I caught my reflection in the car window, and I saw immediately how she viewed me. "Yuck!" Invisible. I had become invisible.

Pre-baby, I had attained a certain level of success in my industry. Becoming a mom at the newly cool age of 42 immediately gave me carte blanche to join the "I don't care how I look now, because I have this beautiful baby" club.

That insensitive woman in the bank line unknowingly redirected my life. That was the day I got a clue.

IT'S NOT OVER YET!

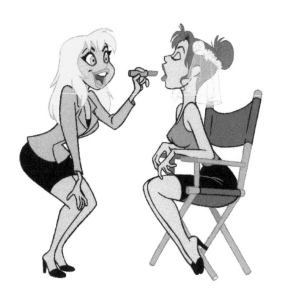

CHAPTER 2

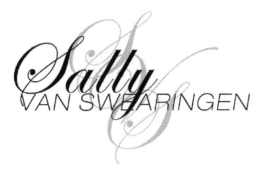

VAN SWEARINGEN

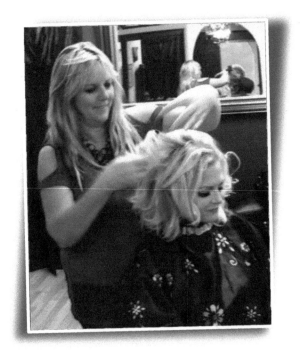

Creating **Beauty Power**
at The A LIST

Mama Knows Some Stuff

Our mama, Eleanore, raised us right. She taught us to get excited about dressing up. "Let's go shopping!" was what we loved to hear our mama say.

Eleanore was a strikingly beautiful blonde Southern woman with natural good looks and amazing cheekbones. She reveled in the experience of getting prepped for an event. Mama made it fun. As soon as we heard the word "shopping," we were ON it. My sister and I would run to the car, excited about the adventure of shopping for new outfits at Bullocks Wilshire or the Broadway. Our mama could shop for hours and was always the last one

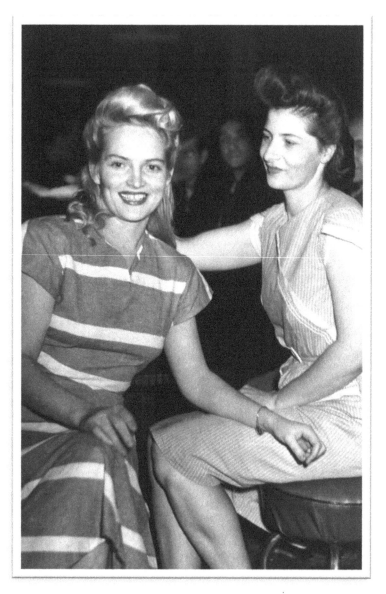

My Mama, Eleanore

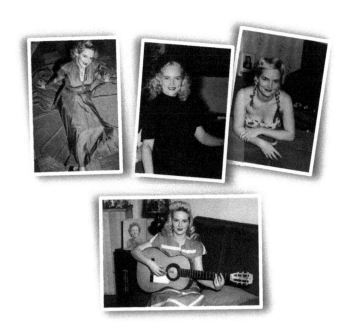

to call it a night. Usually our shopping trips were stimulated by an event we were going to. We had to get our ensembles in order! Dress, shoes, jewelry. She loved clothes and shared her passion for fashion with us by osmosis.

One of my earliest memories is of my mom in a tailored black fitted suit and matching pillbox hat. I was about 6. We were sitting outside of our church and I was staring at her. Her hair was tucked into a chignon and pulled off her face, revealing her true classic beauty.

We had the prettiest mom, yet she seemed unaware of her **Beauty Power.** She had it, and that was clear. Looking through pictures of her and my dad in their younger years was like looking at Hollywood movie stars. We heard it constantly through the years. I do believe our mom's beauty contributed in some way to my career choice.

As our beautiful mama aged, she chose NOT to take advantage of cosmetic surgery procedures that were becoming wildly popular, primarily among the wealthy and celebrity set. My parents were not rich by any means, but they could have afforded these luxuries if my mom so wished.

This was the 1960s and early '70s; stars like Elizabeth Taylor, Phyllis Diller, and Zsa Zsa Gabor were not shy about their procedures. Phyllis Diller included jokes about all of her plastic surgery in her comedy, and it helped to glamorize the plastic surgery industry, later known as cosmetic surgery. With its new name, it didn't sound so ominous. During this time, the idea of going under the knife was still quite scary for many of the mortal population. It wasn't until the 1980s that cosmetic procedures were becoming accepted across the board.

A few years before our beloved mama passed away, she shared with me that she wished she hadn't been so intimidated by plastic surgery, perhaps choosing to have something done that would have made her outside match the way she felt inside. Mama was still striking with her makeup on, yet she felt people viewed her as old when she didn't feel anything of the sort. "When a person starts looking old, they start acting like it," she would say. There are no truer words than those said by my beautiful mother.

Our mama truly believed that a person's reflection in the mirror starts to affect his or her actions. I used to sit on her bed and we would have these talks. "Sally, if you ever feel like it's time to get some procedure done, don't be afraid like I was, just do your homework and get three opinions." I took this advice to heart when I chose to get my eyes done at the age of 48.

After several years of being on my own as a freelance makeup artist, I was choosing to re-enter the salon world. At this same time I was joining the platform speaking industry and producing makeup technique videos. After having my baby daughter at 42, I had begun to look the part of the maxed-out mom, with heavily lidded eyes. I heard, "You look tired" more than I wanted to hear. "NO! I'm NOT tired!" No more than any other mom in her 40s with a young child and a full-time business. I just looked like it!

Gathering Eleanore's wisdom, I interviewed three doctors and found the right one for me. Dr. Babak Azzizadeh listened (more about that later) to my wishes and gave me the conservative look I was after. It works with the rest of my face, and no one could ever guess I had it done unless I choose to tell. But I talk openly about it anyway.

Three days after the procedure (See? Another safe word. "Procedure" sounds so much better than "surgery," which is what it is.) I was on a photo shoot wearing a hat and sunglasses, with the bruises still visible under makeup. People didn't even bat an eye; it's just so common here in Los Angeles. It's almost a status symbol. Before the 1970s it was a carefully guarded secret.

The saying goes: "When we get to the end, it's not the things we DID that we regret. It's what we DIDN'T do."

Life Lesson #2:
Create a Powerful Image

Perception is Powerful

Example A: In the film "Notting Hill," Julia Roberts, who plays a superstar actress who has just garnered another Academy Award, shares with co-star Hugh Grant:

"It's all silly, and none of it is real." Perception is what people believe. I have lived it and know it. As a platform makeup educator, traveling to Toronto and Montreal, I was amazed to hear people in my audience ask me for autographs and pose for pictures with me to hang in their salons. Huh? What did this mean? It meant the marketing worked.

The French Canadian producers of this event had succeeded in convincing this audience that this Los Angeles makeup artist is Hollywood, based on my interactions with celebrities.

Example B: In the 1990s, as a traveling makeup artist with Chanel Cosmetics, I entered my local bank after finishing a gig at a local department store with the Chanel team. The Chanel look was and still is all black from head to toe, a very high-end finish. Flawless makeup and hair. Alfred Hitchcock epitomized this perfected look in his films with his known obsession with cool blondes. That's Chanel.

This day I was completely dressed in the Chanel look. As I entered my bank, the branch manager spotted me and got up from his chair on the opposite side of the expansive room to scoot across the floor and introduce himself. I'm like "Hmm. Uh, I have come in here before, dude." I had the same amount of money in my account that I had the day before, but now I seemed different. I was different. That's perception.

In the film, "Romy and Michelle's High School Reunion," there is a hilarious and thought-provoking theme. In the scenes during which they decide they are going back to their ten-year high school reunion as successful business women, they hadn't

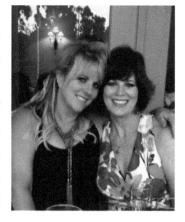

figured yet what business they were actually in, only that they would be entering the party wearing corporate power suits, walking and talking like kick-ass superstars. They knew that if they looked like successful people, they might be perceived as being so. Whether we like it or not, the way we look and act will always affect the way we are perceived.

People treat us as we teach them to treat us.

Let me repeat this for myself, because I had a very tough time learning this one:

PEOPLE TREAT US AS
WE TEACH THEM TO TREAT US

Make it easier on yourself and easier on them. Look the part!

Maturing does an interesting thing to our attitudes about looking the part. Many of us get to a point when we've decided that we don't have to do that anymore. We have earned our place and don't have to dress for the job anymore. I disagree with anyone over 40 who thinks this way.

We never have a second chance to make a first impression.

As I mentioned previously, I can easily pass for a frumpy housewife when I go to my neighborhood grocery store in shorts, a T-shirt and flip-flops. I'm just being comfortable, but to anyone passing by, I'm a mature person who stopped caring and, even worse, is invisible. So WHAT? You may say. Do I have to look like a supermodel going to the store?

I can't tell how many times I made the above mistake and ran into a salon client or, even worse, a potential salon client. Ex-boyfriends are the least of my problems! My reputation and my appearance are my future in this second half of my life.

A quick checklist of Sally Do's to pull it together and look more appealing in minutes:

Apply concealer under the eyes and a dab of lip gloss to your pout (60 seconds).

A little blush wouldn't hurt, too, especially at night when lighting is very unflattering (10 seconds).

Pull on that well-fitting skirt or those cute jeans you feel good in (2 minutes).

Quick spray of tan-in-a-can for those exposed legs— more on this later (60 seconds).

Spray on a spritz of yummy-scented body spray (15 seconds).

I count this little routine as an extra five minutes. A complete natural but polished look has been accomplished.

Feel great and walk proud. You will enjoy your shopping more, you WILL welcome eye contact and maybe even make a new friend or meet your next business contact. Bring it up a notch!

Look the part, and get the part

- Own your weaknesses.

- Recognize your strengths.

- Create the picture.

Rarely do I approach a subject this way, but let's start with the negative! Write down a n y physical characteristics that you believe may prevent you from creating a powerful image.

Why am I asking you to do such a terrible thing? Because it's what people see when they view you, and we must be brutally honest with ourselves if we are going to make a change and rediscover our **Beauty Power.**

Write down what you truly think others see, the way you look and act right now. It doesn't matter here if you agree or not.

Owning your weaknesses:

Are you disorganized, have thinning hair, can't make eye contact, have belly bulge? What do YOU think you are judged on?

_____

_____

_____

_____

Recognizing your strengths:

What's powerful and positive about you?

Perhaps you are a great listener, have stage presence, have nice legs, play drums, make people laugh, have amazing cheekbones, etc.

_____

_____

_____

_____

_____

Create the picture:

What do we want people to see?

Example: "I am a dynamic, fun, skilled, curvy woman who radiates with excitement for what I have to share. I'm happy and self-confident. My life's work is to make women look and feel beautiful. I am a role model. I help others to succeed, and share my life experiences. . I am real, humble and excited about what's next!"

That picture is mine. Now let's do yours.

Let's create a personal Reclaiming My **Beauty Power** "mission statement" from the list of your strengths.

What do we already possess, at this point in our lives, and what do we need to do to have it all?

_____

_____

IT'S NOT OVER YET!

How do you want to be seen?

_____

_____

You may find you are closer than you think.

Create the picture. Write it here.

I,

_____

_____

_____

_____

Now read it back to yourself. It's amazing isn't it? Are you surprised that you already possess so much of what you would like to put out there?

After being truly honest with myself (that's the really tough part), I was able to design my own **Reclaiming My Beauty Power** mission statement. I learned that I need to make three important and solid changes. I wrote down these three changes I must make and committed myself to it.

Sally Must Do #1: Stay Fit.
What's Yours?

I love to eat good food and drink a little wine, but my real weakness is SUGAR! If I didn't have that addiction, I would be slenderer. I LOVE dance, but working out at the gym is a time-sucker. I make myself take dance classes, but as I get busier, I have trouble making it to the gym. My sister Robin is an inspiration.

She and my brother-in-law, Ruben, go five days a week! They fight the aging by working out, and it shows.

Incorporating a buddy system helps motivate. When I realized that I wasn't getting to the gym as much, I self-motivated and re-enrolled in DANCE classes (after a 10-year hiatus) and found some buddies for hiking and walking.

Are you thinking of YOUR must do's? Begin to jot them down here.

_____

_____

Sally Must Do #2: Get a Hearing Aid. What's Yours?

Being hearing impaired most of my life I just dealt with it. During these years, my ego and budget refused to admit I really needed it.

A physical challenge like mine can keep relationships from growing to their best levels. People grow tired of having to repeat themselves and some just stop talking to you altogether! On top of that realization, I think of all the miscommunications that come from it and it boggles my mind. I am doing something about it now. I took proactive steps to find out how impaired my hearing really is and what options are available to me. I'm not going to just live with it anymore. I don't want to miss a thing in my second half.

Is there a physical challenge that keeps you from advancing as fast and as far as you can or causes communication breakdown between you and others around you? At some point, you have to own up to it.

Do you have a physical challenge? If you do, write it here

_____

_____

_____

_____

Do you think this physical challenge is hindering you? How?

_____

_____

_____

_____

What steps will you take to fix it?

_____

_____

_____

_____

Sally Must Do #3: Hire a Clothes Stylist. What's Yours?

Don't stay stuck. For example: I feel confident in black suits, dresses, boots, etc. I think they make me powerful, and it sure is easy to get dressed in the morning! However, others might not view it that way. They might see that I am trying to disguise my figure flaws or just be boring, therefore looking dated and older. That's not good. Let me open myself up to suggestions and take the help of others. Let me gather some more COLOR in my wardrobe.

When I am out shopping for a new outfit, in one of my favorite stores, Cache or Nordstrom, I look for a sales associate who is dressed in something I find interesting; something that I could see myself wearing. If she has a similar body type, then it is even better!

I ask for help in putting together clothes. I find that they pull things I may not have seen or would even have picked up, yet when I put them on, I am often surprised that they work! It is very important to describe your particular taste and preferences to be open to trying something NEW, as long as it is chosen to flatter and not work against your body type. Don't be afraid to immediately reject fashion trends that totally go against your taste. When they start pulling flowery, loose fitting, ethereal clothes for me, I say NO!!! That's not ME.

A great way to get a wardrobe stylist to help you look best is to make a "look book" of fabulous clothes you have seen and that you could imagine yourself wearing. Pinterest.com is a great place to start. Go there now. Check out what women are pinning for themselves. It is addictive, but in a good way. You begin to see how ladies have particular tastes and preferences.

With Pinterest, you can start gathering all the "good stuff" YOU like into one place. Even if right now you don't know what your personal style is, a website like Pinterest is a great place to help you figure it out. Go there, create a profile and start designing yourself! Ask friends, family and acquaintances to follow you. Follow me, too! Here is my link.

www.pinterest.com/sallysstudio/pins

There are lots of fun pictures and good discussion points. It's almost as fun as shopping.

You know the saying: "If you continue to do things the way you always have, things will turn out the same." It's important to get help in this area if you don't want to come home with another navy blue sweater.

Note: *If you wear what you've always worn, you'll look the way you've always looked.*

What clothing items do you repeatedly buy?

_____

_____

_____

_____

_____

_____

Stop the madness! Stop buying those!

How would you describe the personal style you are putting out right now?

_____

_____

_____

_____

_____

What kind of style would you like to have?

_____

_____

_____

_____

_____

It's picture time!

In the space below, paste a photograph of yourself. Choose the last picture of yourself you really liked.

Next, paste a current picture of yourself.

Look at them carefully. What do you see? What has changed?

How do we take the best of the earlier picture and mold it into the design of the new you? What do you love about the earlier you? What part of that would you like to bring forward?

Whether we see it as a positive or negative, Madonna is the queen of reinvention. If you study her, you will see that Madonna has always carried forward the best parts of her authentic look into her next look. As a brand is changing, it evolves to the change.

Keep your best. Change the rest.

What are you keeping about your current look?

_____

_____

_____

_____

_____

_____

What needs to be changed?

_____

_____

_____

_____

_____

_____

Change is very, very hard. Self-acceptance is difficult. But you can achieve it, and you will.

Linnaea Mallette, a speaker, author and role model, is a great example here.

I was brought in to groom the hair and makeup of 57-year-old Linnaea, the hearing-impaired author of "Read My Lips, Tips for Success." She was the keynote speaker at a motivational seminar in L.A. with an audience of 400, which was videotaped in high definition. By now we all know that hi-def can be brutal. A woman with no knowledge of how to prepare to be watched in this technology would be in a bad spot.

Linnaea feels at home in front of an audience, but this was different. She needed to be able to keep them all in eye contact and be relatable to 400 people while still embracing her true self. "Keep the best, lose the rest"

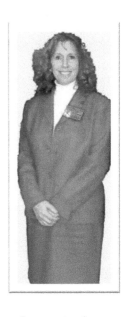

See these pics of Linnaea before and on the day of her keynote. Observe how we keep the best: Linnaea's warm smile, the beautiful curls and red, her signature look.

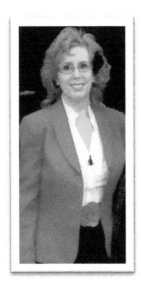

Now we will lose the rest: the dated hairstyle, matronly clothes and nondescript makeup. Linnaea brought in TV wardrobe expert Karen Hudson and ME! She knew this was her moment and she was going to rock it. She did! Here is Linnaea's quote:

"Sally made me look like a movie star when I delivered a keynote at a major marketing event. I mean, I looked BEAUTIFUL. Her products and the techniques for using them made me look younger and healthier. Thank you Sally for helping me rediscover my Beauty Power! You have me for life!"

Love you too Linnaea!

Your notes for change:

_____

_____

_____

_____

_____

_____

_____

_____

_____

_____

_____

_____

_____

_____

_____

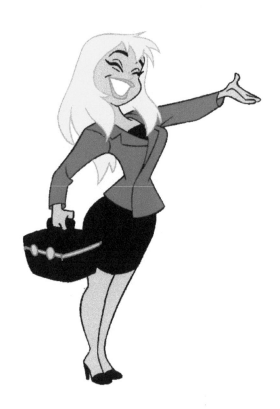

CHAPTER 3

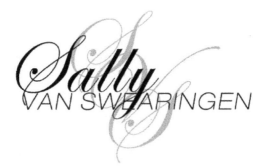

Sally
VAN SWEARINGEN

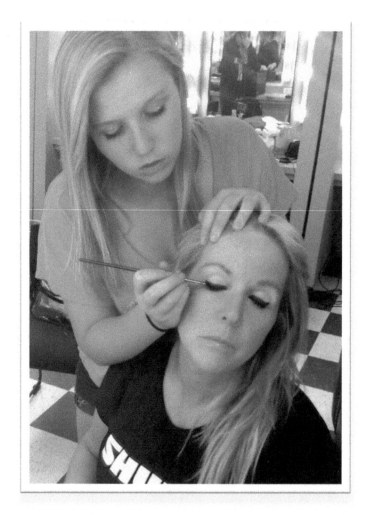

Getting out of my typecast.

Have You Typecast Yourself?

We are well aware of celebrities who have found themselves trapped in the narrow world of typecast. There are scream queens who can get cast only in horror pictures. Child actors who aren't allowed to grow up. Character actors you see only in mafia movies. Do these actors dream of working in different types of projects?

I would guess that most of them certainly would, yet they have been playing a specific role so long that a casting director AND we, the viewing audience, have found a comfort zone in forcing them to repeat themselves incessantly.

As we mature, we each mold an image that seems to stick with us. We think we have changed and evolved, yet we are often stuck in dated thoughts and patterns. We feel secure in our continuity.

We have pictures in our heads of how we think we are supposed to be and pictures of how we think we are coming across. I think all of us should be followed around with a video camera focused on us, capturing our true essence. That would be an eye-opener!

What ROLE have YOU designed for yourself?

Sally's Life Lesson: As we move on in our years, we can lose sight of the fact that we are being judged as much on our maturing age as on all the other issues we might need to address.

My daughter Brigitte is 13 as I write this book. Recently I was thinking that I was a WAY COOL mom when she was entertaining her friends in her room; I checked in four times a night to say hi and hang out for a few. I viewed myself as the fun, connected-to-current-culture mom. I mean, I take popping and locking dance classes! That makes me cool, right? REALITY hit me hard. I'm the creepy old lady who can't stay out of their business and doesn't trust them!

After one too many of my checking-in-to-say-hi room visits, my daughter sarcastically ranted, "Yeah Mom, I'm selling crack to my teddy bears. Can you just STAY OUT?" That was a sobering moment.

Sally, you may be very cool and fun to your friends and your clients, but the 13-year-olds aren't on the same ride. We have to be aware that others view us differently than we see ourselves.

I will never abandon my youthful way of thinking or my desire to be approachable, but for some of us it is absolute that we have a relationship with age-appropriate balance.

There are three extreme types of forty-and-beyond ladies whom I see. This has been my observance both as a forty-and-beyond woman myself and in my profession as a makeup artist and hair stylist.

Hint-hint: You may see yourself here...

Sally's Forty-and-Beyond Woman Typecast #1

Let's call her "Daisy Dukes and Ugg boots Lady."

Oh-my-gosh! I'm getting older! I see lines creeping up around my eyes, my middle is starting to spread and people are calling me "ma-am." I've gotta get to the gym.

OK, cool, I'm working out five days a week now and dieting. I lost another 10 pounds! Looking better, but not good enough. Going to get some new jeans. That will make me feel better.

The designer jeans store in the mall. YES! I can fit into a junior size! All right! Let me get over to Forever 21 (a store for teenagers) and pick up some of those micro short skirts and blingy jeans. I don't care if others think I dress too young. I've got a battle to fight, and I'm going to win.

I gotta stay hot!

It's noon. Can't miss my consult with the cosmetic surgeon. (Cellphone rings.) "Oh, Hi Jennifer! No. I can't have lunch today. I'm dieting. Yes. I'm still on it. Must lose five more pounds. No. I'm NOT eating.

I'm only doing shakes. Yes, I really do miss FOOD. What is it like again? Hmmm... You are having steak and a glass of wine and listening to some jazz? Oh, that sounds so yummy, but I've got to meet up with my personal trainer, we are running the stairs today."

Sally's Forty-and-Beyond Woman Typecast #2

Let's call her "Baseball Cap and Sweat Pants Lady."

Oh-my-gosh! I'm getting older! Wow, looking in this photo album, I see I used to have the looks, didn't I? Man, my legs look tight here! I didn't realize how fit I was. Why was I so hard on myself?

And now here we are, the pictures taken at this past year's Christmas party. Hmm, I have aged. And I sure look thicker too. Oh, well. I'm 46 now, what do I expect? Am I supposed to look like a 22-year- old? That was a long time ago. I'm middle-aged now.

I've got to just accept it. That good-looking, vibrant, athletic girl in the picture? I'm not that person anymore. I'm me: fat, wrinkled and happy.

My husband likes me just the way I am. (Hmm, I wonder if he really feels that way or just doesn't want to hurt my feelings). I mean, I am 30 pounds heavier and have sweats in several colors. But it's nice not having to work so hard, not worrying about waxing my legs, coloring my hair, even putting makeup on. That was such a chore. I'm glad I'm over it.

Those "Botox Barbies" who do all that are just trying to get attention anyway. Hello, honey, we are not teenagers anymore, we have to just let it go.I'm secure with myself. Now, where are those chips? My soap opera is about to start. The ladies on the soaps sure lead the life.

Sally's Forty-and-Beyond Woman Typecast #3

Let's call her "I love My Beauty Power" Lady.

Oh-my-gosh! I'm getting older! Hmm. What can I do to still look good and feel good? The 40s and 50s are NOT a stopping point, they are a starting point! I'm slowly realizing that I can finally do some of the things that I have dreamed of doing and trying. Who is going to stop me? Now I'm getting excited about all of the NEW things I'm going to do with the next part of my life!

It's funny how I resisted yoga and Pilates at first, but it has made such a difference in my body. Now I'm starting to think I don't really miss those brutal aerobics of the 1980s. Why did we do that again?

There's a hiking group starting up. I'm going on Saturday; sounds like the trail they are taking to the waterfall will be beautiful. So my running shoes are turning into hiking shoes. the main thing is to move it, move it!

I love the way my skin feels now that I have re-energized it with facials and products just for me at this time in my life. I don't want to look pulled or fake, I like looking more natural. It's amazing how just a little bronzer or blush works, and I'm shocked that I really don't need all of that makeup! I look younger with so much less.

It's sweet that Natalie's boyfriend says he can see where she got her looks, it was cute to see the grin on her daddy Joe's face. Now, if I can just get Joe to take those ballroom classes with me.

IT'S NOT OVER YET!

Oh! It's noon. Dana and I are sharing pasta today at our favorite Italian eatery while we plan the launch of her new natural soap line. I love having friends who support one another. I didn't even feel like going for a walk last night, but Dana made me get up and do it. I feel good about myself. Wow. I finally got here.

Which of these ladies are YOU? I have been all three of these typecasts, but I aspire to be #3 and I hope you do too.

In this second half of life, which role will YOU be cast in?

How have you typecast yourself?

_____

_____

_____

_____

_____

_____

_____

IT'S NOT OVER YET!

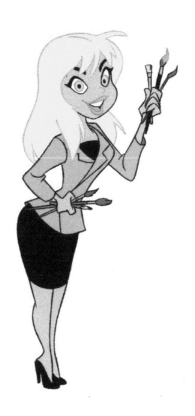

CHAPTER 4

Sally
VAN SWEARINGEN

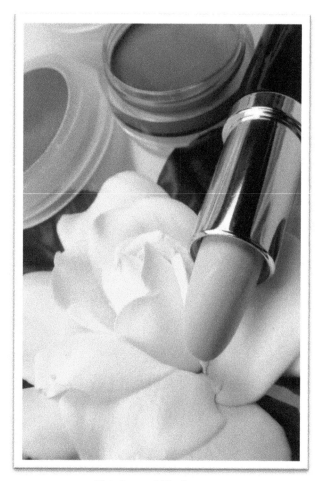

Tricks and Tools.

Bring It Up a Notch: Your Inner/Outer Hottie Beauty Master Plan

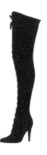

"How to use what you've got to make more of what you are"

I like lists. Lists make me happy and keep me focused.

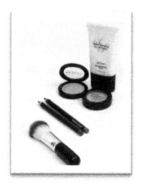

The following is a list for you of all the beauty techniques and tricks that I have personally enjoyed to Reclaim My **Beauty Power.**

"Sally Do" **Beauty Power** Checklist

After reading this list, we will be exploring an expanded description of each.

1. Exfoliation

2. Moisturizer with sunscreen

3. Tinted sunblock

4. BB cream

5. Tinted primer

6. Collagen stimulating night cream

7. Retinol cream

8. Bronzer

9. Cheek and face gleamer

10. Eye area highlighter

11. Neutral lip liner

12. Cream blush

13. Powderliner pencil

14. Lashes

15. Eye shadow primer

16. Lash grow treatments

17. Lash and brow tinting

18. Bangs

19. Velcro rollers

20. Extra hair

21. Shapewear

22. Bras

23. Professional spray tanning

24. Tan in a can

25. Airbrush leg makeup

26. Neutral tone high heels with invisible platform

27. A variety of sexy shoes

28. Opaque black hose

29. Botox (minimally!)

30. Blepharoplasty/brow lift (laser eyelid surgery)

31. Photo facials

32. Rainforest lactic peels

33. Dance classes!

34. Hiking/Walking

35. Yoga

36. Music

37. Radiance through nutrition

38. Sexuality and intimacy/get your playful on

39. Attitude adjustment

Wait a second! You might say. That's a long list! Sounds like you are trying to make me into a Stepford Wives Barbie doll! I don't want to compete with a girl in her 20s or even 30s. I'm experienced, wiser and better for it! I am proud of it.

We are proud. And we are accomplished. And we can still be head turners, in an age-appropriate way. Let me give you an example of where I am going with this.

Think of that ONE lady you know who has soft flowing beautiful silver hair. She probably has an athletic slim build. She works out, you can tell. She may be a yoga teacher or a musician. She is bronzed and healthy looking. She looks GREAT with all of her silver hair and seemingly nonexistent makeup. Maybe you want to try it too. "Heck with it. I'm tired of coloring my hair! I'm going to go grey also."

Really? You are? Are you going to stop wearing makeup too? You might as well just go natural all the way. STOP! That look works for her but, sadly, for very few others. It is the picture she has created for herself, but is it really for you?

Beauty products/professional services/procedures/activities that I credit with helping me to reclaim my Beauty Power

1. Exfoliation: Peel it, peel it.

Youthful skin has an even tone, reflective and luminous, without makeup. Ladies spend millions to duplicate this look with moisturizers, makeup, highlighters and bronzers. This does help, but to REALLY show off our skin we MUST start at the bottom, underneath all the makeup.

At our age, we know how important it is to rid our skin of dead lifeless cells, but are we doing it? With every week that goes by, our skin's natural cell turnover slows down. This can be sped up in several ways:

Salon facials: Salicylic peels and lactic peels are the gentlest way to get the radiance back in the skin. You will need to have a series of treatments and follow them up with hydrating moisturizers and sunblock to truly see lasting results.

At-home scrubs and peels:

Look for pumpkin peels, citrus-based exfoliation products like orange blossom cleansers, and apple pectin-based products. These naturally occurring acids have been used for centuries to naturally smooth the facial skin. The acids break down the uneven, dry upper layer of the epidermis, helping to thin out the aged look of our faces, giving us a more reflective healthy glow.

Even if you have opted for a simple scrub in the shower, you are doing something. Make sure your scrubs dissolve when you use them. Do NOT ever use scrubs that have crushed walnut shells in them. As a licensed esthetician since 1979, I'm shocked that the FDA is still allowing these types of products to be sold in drug stores and large chains. These so-called natural scrubs can cause rashes, burns, cuts and breakouts.

Natural shower scrub: I make a simple in-shower scrub by mixing 1/2 cup of granulated sugar, enough water to make a paste, and a drop of tea tree oil in a small bowl. Tea tree is a natural antibacterial, and the sugar dissolves easily under shower water. So there is really NO excuse for not finding the time or budget to exfoliate.

2. Moisturizer with sunscreen SPF 15-25

For 20 years I have been using a fabulous daily moisturizer that simply has an added SPF 20 sunscreen. It is not a complete coverage but enough to keep unnecessary rays off the skin during the daily activities of driving, walking outdoors briefly, etc. Just using a sunscreen daily of SPF 15 or higher will help keep brown spots and deep lines at bay for several years, and when you do start to see the aging on your face, it will be minimal.

Don't forget your chest and hands. I did often, and as a result my chest doesn't look quite as youthful as my face. Lesson learned!

3. Tinted sunblock

This is another youth saver. Tinted sunblock is a skin-care product that thinks it's makeup. To be a sunblock, a product has to have at least a 30 SPF of both UVA and UVB rays. The warm, peachy color in the creamy zinc-based product gives an instant coverage, great for ladies on the go who need the extra coverage but don't want to feel smothered in greasy sun block.

4. BB cream

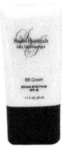 BB Cream is the beauty industry's push product as of the writing of this book. Every major cosmetic company is pushing its own BB cream. What is it? BB stands for beauty balm. It's an all-inclusive product, and the best single product for many purposes. Lighter in consistency

than a tinted sunblock, BB cream is a sunblock, foundation, moisturizer and treatment cream all in one. Toss it in your purse. It is a must-have to slow your skin's aging from the sun.

5. Tinted primer

Tinted primer is an excellent example of new technology and how our maturing skin will benefit from it! This product is light and slightly luminous. Lighter than foundation, it goes on the skin to create a very smooth canvas. Be sure to use one that contains sunblock, and toss that foundation that is probably making your skin look older!

6. Collagen stimulating night cream

You don't have to load your skin down with heavy creams, but you must keep the facial skin nurtured while you sleep. We do a lot of our perspiring at night. This means more moisture loss. When we wake in the morning, we wonder why our skin looks so dry and the lines are more visible. It has been proven that a potent collagen stimulating cream will actually deep-moisturize parched aging skin by reenergizing collagen threads in the dermis and epidermis, strengthening the bonds that keep skin pliable and younger looking.

If I am just too lazy to do anything else, I try at least to quickly cleanse my face and put on my night cream. If I haven't done it, my makeup does not look so good the next morning. When I am working on set as a makeup artist, there is nothing more challenging than to try to brighten up on-camera talent when they are lacking sleep and haven't used a night cream. Ladies, it is vitally important to keep your skin extra moist! People ask me why my skin isn't deeply lined. I am convinced that my years of taking an extra minute to apply facial cream has its rewards.

7. Retinol cream

Retinol cream is a Vitamin A-based resurfacing cream. This type of product works wonders on maturing, sun-damaged and blemished skin. It's a good product to share with your hormonal–acned teenager! Retinol cream increases the production of cells in the top layer of skin, helping to rejuvenate the skin. As a result, the skin gradually looks younger. The cream also promotes more collagen production, making the skin appear plumper. It may also reduce pigmentation issues that stem from sun damage. Be aware that you will become sun-sensitive, so always use a sunblock when using retinol. Your doctor can give you a prescription for a medical grade cream, but I would start with an over-the-counter level, which won't be as strong. By now you may have figured me out. I take the conservative approach to anything chemical! It is always better to err on the side of caution when it comes to chemicals and skin care.

8. Bronzer

Bronzer is one of the most important beauty products a forty-and-beyond woman needs in her arsenal. When it is applied correctly bronzer brings a natural looking youthfulness to the face and décolleté, (chest area). It is an absolute essential for my personal daily use, especially for photographs. Bronzer helps me get a sharper and more prominent jawline. Salon clients get completely jazzed when I show them how to become experts at using their magic wand.

My product, Studio Essentials Bronze Goddess, is shown to all my new clients because it is easy and quick, and it instantly warms the complexion. Choose a cream-based or powder bronzer and apply it under the cheekbones along the jawline, on the chest and at the top of your face at your hairline to create an oval effect. Light to medium skins need a soft coral-bronze, darker skins need more orange red-based color. Darkest skins need red-orange.

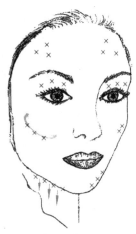

To see a video showcasing the use of the bronze pencil, go to **www.SallyVanSwearingen.com**

9. Cheek and face gleamer

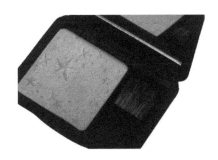

As a freelance makeup artist, I am a part of a few production teams. These teams are hired to go on location to shoot in-house promos, launches, interviews, commercials, etc. for corporate clients.

Deep Image Productions, was filming at Guess headquarters in Los Angeles. We were shooting interviews with CEO Paul Marciano and Guess department heads. One of the big bosses, who was in her mid- to late 50s, took her spot in front of the camera. I stepped in and quickly added a

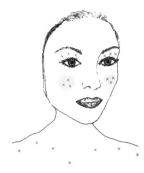

luminizing, gleaming blush to her cheeks and eyes. The crew actually gasped at the transformation. The director, while looking at the monitor, asked me, "What did you just do to her? You made her look 10 years younger!" I told him it was a new product that you can get online. I didn't want to say it was MY own product, but it was! A few of the ladies who were on set that day got online and ordered it, because they saw with their own eyes what a product like that can do.

As we age, we tend to lose the fullness in our upper faces, the rounded cheek area of youth starts to thin out. Simply applying a gleaming type of product on the apples of the cheeks (while smiling) gives the illusion of roundness, therefore making a woman's face look more youthful.

10. Eye area highlighter

Take the TIRED look away.

I am amazed and surprised that I don't see more makeup artists using this technique for their on-camera work. I learned a great trick when I started out, landing a spot as an assistant at the Long Beach Civic Light Opera. I watched the makeup artists apply a white cream at the top of the cheekbone and at the brow line of each of the actors. It really made their eyes stand out, even if you were sitting many rows back. I took this intense stage makeup technique and made it more natural for my brides by using an eggshell-colored cream stick in those areas. For darker complexions, I simply use a more amber-toned shade. I've been doing this for years, and it has become one of my signature makeup tricks.

To see this and the products being demonstrated, check out my "Beauty Power" Video on www.SallyVanSwearingen.com

11. Neutral lip liner

When we think of natural beauty it usually includes a subtle lip color. A neutral lip pencil can do amazing things for a woman's mouth, whether you have my issue (small lips) or lips fuller than you would like. (OK, seriously, do very many woman

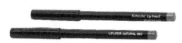

actually have that problem??) I often use a neutral lip liner to base the lips and round out the shape. We can believably make the mouth look about 20% fuller with this technique. I am a real stickler for properly shaping the mouth. If you create the most beautiful makeup but improperly shape the mouth, the entire face will be off balance. One of the first areas where we begin to see aging in the face is the upper lip, which begins to thin and flatten. However, this is one of the easiest and most dynamic

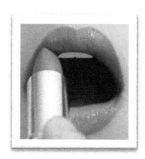

corrections we can make, and it gives immediate results. Try this: With a neutral pencil, round out the top of the lip, slightly cheating above and beyond the natural line. This can only be ever so slight. More conservative rounding will give you a more believable result. Then follow your natural lip shape, slightly rounding again at the bottom. Let's have art class for a minute. Get a red apple and watch how the light hits it. See how the light is stronger at the top and the base (bottom). This is how to properly shape the lips.

To see a video demonstrating this technique go to
www.SallyVanSwearingen.com

12. Cream blush

Blush in general is underused by women in the second half! Cream blush is an amazing product to bring out the cheekbones and give a soft rounded look to the apples of the cheeks. Creams tend to look more natural and stay put longer than powders. Creams keep skin looking moist, which is vital to youthful appearing skin.

Cream blush, once known as rouge has been around since the 1920s. There is no other cosmetic item that is so versatile and flattering. As a makeup artist, I can do a lot with one pot of this miracle maker. Cream-based blushers and shadows are much more forgiving on the skin than their powder- based counterparts. Creams tend to

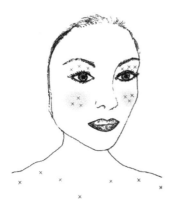 sit on top of the skin and are more easily blended to enhance one's own features. My opinion is that cream blushes tend to be misunderstood by the user and do require a little more time to perfect. The universally most flattering and age-defying shade is a

warm based peachy bronze color. In other words, if I can choose one tone, I will go warm, not cool. Examples: peach, not pink; red-orange, not blue-red. The level of color of course depends on your particular skin tone.

Using your fingers, apply your cheek color on the apple of the cheek, starting on the underside of the cheekbone.

Put most of your application there and then blend it onto the full apple, smiling while you apply, to determine exactly where your apples are. A classic makeup artist trick is to brush a stroke of cheek color on your eyelids to brighten them up.

13. Powderliner pencil

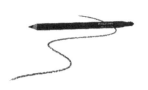 I got hooked on powderliner pencils a long time ago, and rediscovered them when I noticed my regular oil-based pencils not lasting and moving around too much. Powderliners stay in place better and are more forgiving on our eyes. They are easy to blend, using the little sponge tip applicator and are especially great for ladies who have trouble with standard liner pencils.

14. Lashes

Pick up a magazine right now. If you see a celebrity or model on the cover, you can bet she is most probably sporting faux (false) eyelashes. Lashes open up the eyes, making them look huge on camera and in photographs.

FYI: I would never consider having my picture taken or being on camera without lashes.

The first step is to determine which type of lashes are the most flattering to your eye shape and your total look. The most natural and conservative look is individual lash clusters, applied at the outside corners of the eye. Usually about six on each side will 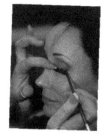 do the trick. I recommend having a professional show you how to do it, because it will require some practice. Do NOT decide to put on your lashes for the first time on the day of an important event! If you have a steady hand, you can apply your own lashes. Take several individual lashes out of the package, using the underside on your thumb.

Place them on top of your opposite hand or on a paper towel.

Using tweezers, pick up a lash from middle point, facing out, as it would lie on the lash line. Dip each lash into lash glue. One dot is enough. Start at the outside edge and work in. Do the right eye first, then the left, with each lash, so you will achieve a balanced look. By the time you get to the iris of the eye, you should have achieved the effect you are seeking.

If you are into a more dramatic look, a complete lash strip is for you.

My favorite is the 747s by Ardell. A makeup friend has worked with Michelle Pfeiffer for her film roles and always used the 747s on her. These are a popular choice for film and TV because they look the most natural from the side and straight on, and that's why I choose them most often for my brides.

Another good choice is the spiky style lash; often called the Liza lash, because it is what Liza Minnelli, Cher, Christina Aguilera, Lady Gaga and many other performers choose as a signature lash because it has a mod, edgy look and makes eyes look huge on camera.

Lash strips also require a little work, but they are worth the effort. You will have to trim them from the outside edge to match the length of your eye, not every lash strip automatically fits every eye! Once that is done, you can usually wear them about three times, and they actually fit the eye better the second time.

Apply glue along the lash line very sparingly, using a dot more at the inner and at the outer eye. Wait about 15 seconds to allow the glue to get a bit sticky, then apply, putting the pressure on the middle of the lash, then gingerly pressing the sides. You may glue your eyes together for a second; don't freak out, it is not permanent! Just gently separate. If the lashes still just don't fit right, trim them a bit more, always from the outside edge. You will get the hang of it with practice, I promise.

Salon Lash Extensions: Although pricey, lash extensions done at a salon can be very beautiful and so flattering to the eye. These are individual lashes, longer than your natural lash, that are carefully applied to your own lash with permanent glue. The process can be tedious for the esthetician and time-consuming for you, but in most cases the results are worth the effort. You can sleep, shower and live in these lashes, but they still do require some maintenance. As your own lashes come out, so will these extensions, and they will require replacing as they do. They typically last a couple of months, but lifestyle and personal care make the difference.

The initial investment can be around $300, so get testimonials and referrals from happy clients before you proceed.

I have asked several ladies what their experience has been. Most LOVE the look, but not the care, maintenance and cost. Some feel relying on lash extensions as a permanent beauty staple can wreak havoc on their natural lashes. This is where "everything in moderation" is key. Lash extensions are a luxury treat, not a permanent solution.

15. Eye shadow primer

The #1 question my salon clients ask is how to make their eye shadow last all day. A shadow primer or shadow magnet has double benefits: It smooths the eyelid to the brow line into one light tone and then keeps the eye color in place all day. A must-have beauty essential!

Why do makeup artists insist on using shadow primer every time?

Shadow primer acts like a magnet for eye shadow, keeping it exactly in its place for hours. Eye shadows go on smoothly and evenly and resist smudging. You don't get that crease in the lid as much as you would without using it. As we mature, our lids need extra help keeping that pretty color on the eyes. Shadow primer to the rescue! Choose a primer in a tone that blends easily with your skin color, whether light, medium or deep.

16. Lash grow treatments

Revitalash: I have used the brand Revitalash to strengthen and grow my lashes. This stuff works, but only if you remember to apply it often. Developed by an ophthalmologist, it is a serum that is absorbed by the skin and stimulates growth. Apply it once per day along the lash line. It retails for about $100 to $150

Latisse: This product is a prescription product that stimulates lash growth and can be purchased through your dermatologist or at a medi-spa. It works but is pricey. It retails for about $200.

17. Lash and brow tinting

About ten years ago, I took the best makeup class I ever had! It was given at the MAC makeup store in Los Angeles by Sam Fine, the amazingly talented and much loved makeup artist, who has made his name as a makeup guru for women of color. His clients include Queen Latifah, Tyra Banks, Iman, supermodels and many other high-profile ladies. Whether you are a woman of color or not, I would recommend his book, "Fine Beauty."

Sam set up his model and went to work, showcasing his skills with highlighting and shading. He was such a down-to-earth guy and so open about his techniques and tools. Some makeup artists can tend to hold back their secrets, but Sam wasn't like that.

He specifically pressed on the subject of brow and lash tinting. Sam showed us that by simply changing the depth of color on a woman's brows, we can make a significant impact on the dynamic of a face shape.

For instance, blondes have lighter brows. As we mature, the brows become sparser and the color will usually go even lighter or will be mixed with gray, a sign of aging! Tinting the brows slightly darker, in a medium brown shade, brings out every single hair. We need every eyebrow hair, ladies! The brow line becomes more prominent, therefore lifting the upper face. I tint my brows a medium brown shade about every six weeks, and it immediately gives my face a stronger look. This is an absolute must for ladies with light skin and light eyebrows. People will take notice. Your eyes are dominant again!

On the other hand, let's say you have very dark brows, dark hair and a sculpted, strong bone structure. With maturing, this combination can make a woman look hard. Lightening the color of the brow to a soft brown opens up the eyes so the face takes on a softer, more feminine look.

Our lashes can also become sparser with age. Sorry, ladies, I hate to be the bearer of so much bad news, but these are truths. The good news is, I have solutions!

Tinting the lashes black with a blue or violet undertone makes every lash pop and helps counteract some of the redness in the eyes. When you apply mascara, you don't have to work so hard, as the base of the lashes is already dark.

Book an appointment with your esthetician today. Be sure she uses a vegetable dye, which is non-caustic.

These simple beauty tricks can make a subtle but prominent difference in your **Beauty Power.**

18. Bangs

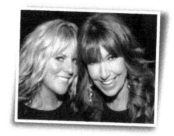

At my studio we have catchy saying: "Bangs or Botox." Bangs give the face an amazing lift. All of a sudden there are cheekbones, and the eyes look huge!

I'm not suggesting short, cut-across-the-forehead bangs, I'm talking about face-framing bangs and those that are angled and longer, like skimming the brow line. If your hair is very curly or wiry, then bangs are not for you unless you do a chemical straightening.

I have a client, Connie, who has naturally curly hair and loves to wear it that way but also loves the look of bangs, so she chooses to have only her bangs professionally relaxed, so she can wear an edgy, current style in her bangs, yet still show off her sexy curly hair. Go for it, Connie!

I will suggest bangs when I know the client will take the time to at least blow-dry them. Bangs look beautiful when styled

---

Styling Tip: use a larger round brush to create a smooth, almost straight look to your bangs, a medium round brush to give a curve to the bang. Slowly pull the brush downward and hold for a couple of seconds at the bottom, this will keep all the length in the bangs, while giving the finished look you are going for. Try both styles to see what best suits you and your beauty regime.

---

19. Velcro rollers

Everything old is new again! Velcro rollers are seriously our BEST friend, girls. What is a Velcro roller? These are large, 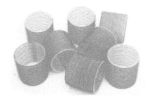 light plastic rollers covered with a Velcro-type material, that, when put in the hair, will stay put.

You can find these rollers at your beauty supply or larger retail outlet. Every single new client in my chair is introduced to the magic of Velcro rollers. At first they may look at me like "Oh no, that's too complicated, I'm not doing that! I don't have time, blah blah blah." Let me tell you: Velcro rollers actually save you time when getting your **Beauty Power** going in the morning. Velcro rollers create a memory in your hairstyle that with proper finishing will stay many hours.

I did grooming makeup for a series of interviews on the "Desperate Housewives" set. Between filming, the gorgeous "housewives" were all in Velcro rollers. On major fashion shoots and runway shows, the rollers remain in the hair right up until show time. If they are good enough for supermodels and "Desperate Housewives," they are OK for us too!

Start by putting a volumizing mousse in the hair when it is still wet. One of my favorite products to use is Guts by Redken. Dry your hair almost completely. Use a medium round brush on the top and sides. By the way, Velcro rollers are an excellent cheat tool for those of us who don't always do a proper salon blow-dry on our hair. You can get the hair basically dry, blow out the front with a round brush and use the rollers to create the rest of the style.

Once the hair is dried, section the crown of your hair by parting it in a V shape (see photos). Then arrange the rollers on the top of your head in a triangular shape.

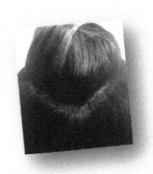

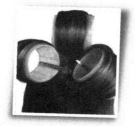

Then all of the other rollers follow suit, being careful to roll them forward and slightly

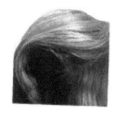

off the base, so that when they come out you get a C shape, lifted effect. Once in place, lightly spray with a working hair spray, not a finishing or strong spray, as that will make the rollers stick and hard to remove. Adding a little extra heat will lock the curl into the style for a longer set. Let sit for at least five minutes; 15 minutes is even better. When you gently remove them, all you need to do is finger through your style. Do not brush. Another quick spray and you are out the door! Gorgeous. **Beauty Power!**

20. Extra hair

As we mature, many of us find that our hair has thinned, and we can't grow our hair as long as we would like. It grows to little points at the bottom, resulting in a straggly appearance. Many of us have husbands who prefer us with long hair, but it simply doesn't

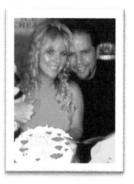

work for us when we try to get it past our shoulders and still looking full, sexy and healthy.

Sorry, guys, but when our hair will not grow past our shoulders without looking damaged, it is time to make a decision: cut it shorter, blunt at the bottom and layered, OR add some extra hair.

Writing about extra hair makes me smile, because it brings me back to 2005, when the stylists at Expose Salon helped me get my hottie back. I had recently lost about 20 pounds and was feeling pretty good. You know that feeling when all your clothes are looking new again and you have a newfound relationship with shopping. I went shopping for hair!

Previously, I had experimented with hair extensions, but I found them to be unnatural looking; they left me with stripper hair. At my age, that look just didn't work. On vacation in Cabo San Lucas, swimming in the pool, my man teased me about my "Frankenstein" hair, because my sewn-in extensions had started to unravel and were hanging on the side of my head! I vowed to be done with the hair extension relationship.

Then, about a year later, our family relocated to Valencia, Calif., and I moved my business into a local salon. I watched for months as ladies with very natural looking, gorgeous new hair left the salon. I soon learned the keys to undetectable extra hair:

- The quality of the hair
- The correct shades to match your own hair and show dimension
- The stylist doing the work.

When I wear my extensions, they are the Hair Locs method, which are individual clusters of hair strands attached to your own hair. You have to commit to some special hair care, like pulling it back at night or braiding it. You also can't brush through it from the roots, as you would your own hair, but in every other way it looks REAL. Very few people ever guess it is not all mine. EVERYONE knows, but only because I tell them.

Celebrity Anecdote

The first season of the TV show "Gossip Girl," I was working on set, doing promos for the new fall lineup for NBC. Blake Lively was a gorgeous up-and-coming actress. On the set she fretted a bit about her extensions and said she was having them taken out. Would I be careful that they looked okay in the shot? They were using a studio fan, so this was a slight challenge. I had to do a little "MacGyver" work to make sure they didn't show themselves, but she looked incredible. See, ladies? Even celebrities have their hair extension hassles.

How to Choose:

Types of Extensions:

- Wefts (or tracks)

- Individual beaded

- Taped In

Wefts

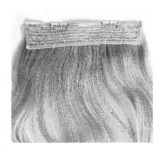

Weft clip-ins are great for a night out and special occasions. They are easy to use and are the least damaging to your hair in the long run. I would suggest trying clip-ins for your first hair extension experiment. Be sure to get hair that matches your own color. It is a good idea to bring a friend with you to help determine the correct shade. Make sure you get enough, as the easiest way to spot fake hair is to see the thinner-looking long pieces that don't match the thickness of your natural hair. Google hair extensions in your area and find a large store that carries a variety. Always buy REAL hair and get the BEST hair your budget allows. The cheaper the quality of hair, the less time the hair will look natural. If you are honestly going for one or two times of use, inexpensive is fine, but don't try to make cheap hair look like part of you.

Sewn-in wefts are the type I had the first time. They looked amazing at my 30-year high school reunion. People really didn't suspect it wasn't all my own hair, and hair IS a guy magnet. I felt pretty gorgeous that night, and my man couldn't keep his hands off me. The downside is that they didn't stay looking great for long.

Wefts are best suited for those with naturally thicker hair and for those who want really big hair, Beyonce style. Wefts are the highest maintenance of all hair extensions, so get ready to spend a good amount of money with your hair stylist to keep them looking real. I have seen some great-looking weft work on actresses and models. And will I use them again? Probably, but only for a big night out. I will not try to get away with it looking like my own hair. BTW, do you think all those Victoria's Secret hotties have their own hair? NOT.

Individual beaded

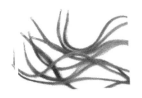

Individual beaded is the type I wear now. As I mentioned above, they are individual bunches of hair attached to a flat titanium or plastic bond and attached to your own hair in rows, as few as one or two and as many as four or five, depending on the length and thickness desired. Every few months you will need to have hair maintenance. Hair that has become less smooth is replaced with newer pieces. They are also moved up on your head. As your own hair grows, the positions of the extensions move. I wear a full set of extensions for as long as 18 months, then take them all out for about six months. The damage to the hair is minimal, as long as you see your stylist regularly for maintenance. Wearing individual extensions takes some training and commitment. You cannot just brush through your hair the way you normally would. You have to grip the hair at the base and brush only through the length. I recommend investing in some light oil, such as Macadamia oil. Apply a few drops to your hands and work through the ends on dry hair. This trick keeps the hair smoother and blended into your own.

At night you MUST tie it into a loose Scrunchy or braid it. This keeps the hair in place while you sleep and keeps tangles at bay. My opinion is that individual beaded-in extensions look the most natural, lie on the head nicely and hold up the longest, with careful attention.

Taped-in

The newest type of extensions is taped in. These are a cross between clip-in type temporary extensions and individual beaded ones. Taped-in can last longer with care and, because they are flat, they fall against the head in a more 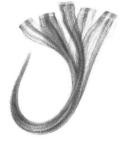 natural way than clip-ins. DO NOT try these extensions by yourself the first time. It could be a disaster, and you would be cussing me out for suggesting them to you.

The benefits? They hold on better than clip-ins, don't move, are more undetectable and can be removed easily by a professional. They are literally taped to your hair close to the scalp. To remove, they are gently pulled off after applying a removing solvent. I suggest going to a reputable salon to have them put in and removed. You will thank me later!

21. Shapewear

Choosing the right shapewear makes you love your curvy body again

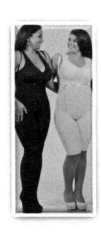 A call came in earlier this year. It was from a friend who is one of my favorite photographers, Emad Asfoury of LA Color Studio. He wanted to book me for a shoot. Cool. I was to find out that he wasn't calling me for make-up and hair. He wanted to pay me to MODEL! Wow, that is very cool!

He explained that his client was looking for voluptuous women who wanted to be just a little more Kim Kardashian-ish.

What a fun experience to be photographed in Elsa's Curves, a new shapewear product.

This hottie-maker product really worked! It's more comfortable than most and does give you that hourglass figure. Once I got myself in it, with some assistance, I was amazed at the way my black slightly fitted dress fit differently. My waist was definitely smaller, hips in balance.

What I DON'T like about a lot of shapewear is how it pushes everything around and makes you look oddly shaped, and of course you can't breathe or sit. The entire evening you are looking forward to just taking it off! I can hear a hairstylist friend saying to us girls in the salon a few years ago, "OK, it's time. I need to go remove my shape wear. I can feel my organs shutting down." Hilarious but true! Can we relate? Elsa's Curves is actually semi-comfortable. I can see myself wearing her garment to a party for the evening. This may sound like an infomercial, but this was my actual experience.

These garments are compression shapewear. Elsa was a nurse's aide who worked with cosmetic surgery patients following their tummy tucks and liposuction procedures. She learned how wearing shapewear immediately after surgery helps recurve the body. Her grandmother also believed in binding the waistline to keep it small. This mind-set is what created Elsa's Curves.

For information on this product contact me at
Sally@ItsNotOverYet.net

What to look for in choosing shapewear:

- Shapewear should NOT be uncomfortable.

- Shapewear should be of a lighter, moldable material.

- Shapewear should NOT contort your body.

I recommend starting with a bodysuit, (similar to a one piece bathing suit), with which you can wear your own bra. Trying to find a bodysuit to fit you correctly, do its' job to shape you and properly lift and shape your breasts is almost impossible, but not completely.

Don't Cheap Out!

This is one item that you need to be willing to invest some good money in. You get what you pay for. Nordstrom is an excellent place to start your search. They have associates who will measure you for a perfectly fitting bra and find you the correct garment for your body type and figure concerns. I purchased a bodysuit at Nordstrom, at the time I thought was way overpriced, yet it served me well for several years and was worth the investment.

My favorite one now is an affordably priced bodysuit from Maidenform. It can be purchased at JC Penney, Kohl's and Macy's. You wear your own bra with it. I have a black one and a flesh-colored one. Be sure to have both.

Many ladies go to a local store and start trying on all kinds of flesh-binding garments, not really knowing what they are looking for. You must get some assistance in this area. Do not go it alone. You may want to call ahead and book a fitting appointment, so all the attention is on you. Bring the garment you plan to wear with it, along with slips, bras, etc.

Size matters, but not this time!

You may be a size small from one manufacturer and a large from another. All that matters is that your garment smooths you and flatters you without causing bulges in other places. Take photographs of yourself from the front, side and back in your garment, wearing your shapewear. You know what they say about a picture and the truth it tells. Make sure the garment hasn't flattened your breasts once you put on the dress or pushed your extra boob flesh into another area.

If you feel you can take it, get an honest friend to assess the final look. But the most important thing is how you feel when you put it on. If you can move, sit and walk comfortably and it makes you feel sexy, you have chosen the right shapewear for your figure.

As my mama used to say, "If you feel good in it, strut!"

22. Bras

As I mentioned above about shapewear, it is vital that you have the properly fitting bra and are sized by a professional. You may say "Duh. Oprah told us all that long ago. Tell me something I don't know."

Here is what you may NOT know about bras:

- Before bras came along, women simply bound their breasts with fabric to flatten them. It was not until the post-1930s that the idea of projecting the breasts came into fashion.

- If you are interested in fact finding, it is an adventure to figure out WHO actually invented the first bra, because there are a lot of speculation and inventors taking credit. What I do know is that the Greeks bound their breasts for battle (as when we wear sports bras!) and later several varieties of breast supports were tried. Maidenform was one of the first companies to give actual shape to the breast without compressing it.

Depending on the size and shape of your breasts, garments from certain manufacturers may be better suited for you. This is why going to a fitting will benefit you. The professional fitters know their manufacturers and can direct you right to the most flattering and best-fitting garment, based on your shape, size, the amount of lift you want to achieve, etc.

Most ladies wear too large a band width and too small a cup size.

Bras lose their effectiveness with age. Depending on how many bras you own, you should replace your bras every year and get re-measured, especially if you have lost or gained weight.

Bras with too much spillage actually make you look older, not sexier. If you are fuller-breasted, you need the fit to be wide at the sides, smoothing that area. This will also help to direct breasts forward. Wider straps will make your clothes fit better and smoother in the shoulders and you won't have that dig that instantly screams that a bra is too small for the big boobies. Last, the properly fitted bra for fuller-breasted women is wide and smooth and across the back. Please, no back fat, ladies!

Small-breasted ladies need pushups too, especially after 40 and children. Pads can be removable. A well-constructed bra is also important here. Some petite ladies can tend to pick flimsy bras that may look sexy to the eye but do nothing to enhance and volumize the breast. When you are being fitted, explain how you would like your breasts to look. Naturally shaped? Pushed up high? More cleavage? All this needs to be discussed. I am loving the new natural look and feel to the inserts for bras these days. Bras with a little extra help are very flattering if your breasts have lost some of their perkiness. Take advantage of all the technology and the millions of dollars that has been spent on the research and development of bras that help you get your **Beauty Power** back!

The bra you wear while exercising needs to be a sports bra, not your clothes bra! You need support at the top, sides and bottom for any activities that involve jumping, running and bouncing.

I recommend removing your bra every night, giving your breasts freedom from compression for several hours, allowing time for free blood flow everywhere around the breast tissue. I'm sure your honey will like it too. It is said that Marilyn Monroe wore a bra to bed every night to keep her breasts from sagging. C'mon people, does that even sound like Marilyn?? I say NOT!! Sleeping with a bra does not keep your breasts supple. However, exercising with the correct, properly supportive bra does.

What do I know about undergarments?

I have been on set enough times to see many a celebrity fitted by a wardrobe stylist with shapewear and a properly fitted bra.

> Bottom line shapewear is not just for women who have figure challenges. Shapewear is to bring out your best figure.

23. Professional spray tanning

I was fortunate to be chosen to be on the makeup team for "Booty Firm," an exercise/dance product infomercial hosted by Mark Ballas, and supported by Maksim Cherkovskiy and Kym Johnson; "Dancing with the Stars" on ABC. These are some of the

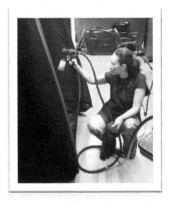

hardest- working people! They have to make it look easy, take after take. Our job as makeup and hair stylists is to help all of the dancers keep looking smooth and perfect.

One beauty inclusive that makes our work as makeup artists so much easier for on-camera beauty is spray tanning. Spray tanning the legs, arms and torso gives the body a tanned appearance, yes, but there is so much more to it. An overall uniformity of tone gives the body a more elongated look. Spray tanning helps to cover bruising and varicose veins and makes brown spots and other unsightly skin issues not as obvious. It brings out the shape of the muscles; even if you aren't built like a professional dancer. As former Las Vegas showgirl Lori Hall says, "Tanned fat looks better!"

A spray-tanned belly makes it look that much leaner. Many salons offer spray tanning services; ours does! Spray-tanning artists can perform body-enhancing miracles. Our local tanning artist totes a cute little mobile booth into the salon, has you get naked and tans you up.

The manually sprayed cooling mist makes several passes on your back, legs, torso, you get the picture. My artist takes special care to get an even color, something you can't get in a stand- up spray-tanning booth. I ask her to make my tummy darker, because I think it looks slimmer, so I'm happier. Spray-tanning professionals can also do creative embellishments, like carving six packs on your abdomen, making the flanks a slightly darker shade to get a slimmer, longer line and, my favorite, contouring away any extra knee fat. The point is, make friends with your local tanning artist!

How long does spray-tanning last? Exfoliating before spray tanning gives a cleaner, smoother look and using lots of moisturizer after the procedure keeps the tan longer. My experience has been four days to a week, depending on the depth of care. Many celebrities who have the budget for it have it done weekly.

Tip: Don't take a shower for several hours after your spray- tan. The next day and days after, take quick showers and don't scrub any tanned areas. Don't rub hard when drying; pat dry instead of rubbing and apply moisturizer right away. Keep moisturizing always!

---

24. Tan in a can

Spray tanning in a can, like Neutrogena (my favorite), temporarily stains the skin and can last up to a week. It's affordable (about $13 a can) and great if you are in a crunch. Got white legs and need help immediately? Tan in a can to the rescue. The downside is that it's always challenging to get smooth, even coverage. Less is always more when building up to the color you want, especially on the back of the legs and arms. However, it is great to have on hand for emergencies. I always carry a can with me when I travel. Be sure to put it in your suitcase, not your carry-on. I learned that lesson when mine was confiscated at check in!

25. Airbrush leg makeup

Airbrush leg makeup can be purchased at your local drug store. The spray cans usually give you about three applications. Leg makeup is different from tan in a can. Airbrush makeup is an actual foundation base makeup that is put into a mist-able form. It is for one use and washes off in the shower. Beauty queens count airbrush leg makeup as one of their staple items. Because it is an actual makeup for the body, airbrush makeup gives the skin a smooth, even tone and covers light bruising, discoloration and varicose veins. It looks natural on camera too, whereas tan-in-a-can tends to look shiny and a bit patchy. The challenge is getting even coverage. Spray a light coat and let it dry, then do another.

Let's say it's getting warm outside, spring has arrived! It's not quite time to be sporting tan legs, but your legs haven't seen the sun in months; and it's brutally obvious! Your skin is uneven in color and you consider putting that cute dress back in the closet.

You don't want to actually look tan yet, but dull winter skin is unattractive! This is when you grab your leg makeup and spray it on. Start with one light coat and let dry. As we mature, our legs get less colorized. Have you ever noticed that? Always choose the warmest shade you can find that will match your skin tone.

Look in the mirror. Does it blend with the rest of your skin? If so, it can be sprayed a little more heavily on areas that need more attention. Be sure it dries thoroughly before attempting to sit, cross legs or rub against anyone. It will wash off in the shower, so DO NOT wear it with your bathing suit unless you are competing in the Miss USA pageant.

26. Neutral-toned high heels with invisible platform

On the set, one wardrobe essential that is usually present if a woman's legs are revealed: neutral- or taupe- toned stilettos with

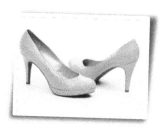

an invisible platform in the shoe.

A neutral tone shoe makes the legs look longer; they don't break up the line the way a black pump or colored one does, especially on camera. The line of the leg continues. I learned this from wardrobe stylists years ago, and they have been a key item in my show wardrobe, in the neutral tones, ever since. The invisible platform, inside the shoe, sets the bottom of the foot up higher, giving a woman a natural-looking inch taller leg.

A No-No: Ladies, the overly platformed extremely high heels, which are in style now and are in our faces everywhere, do not work for us over-40 girls. There are several brutally obvious reasons, but let me state just two:

- It's challenging to walk in a natural, womanly sway in these shoes. It is more like Frankenstein, hobbling along, trying to avoid falling down and breaking a leg. Our facial expression says "This is NOT comfortable."

Is that sexy? No. Young ladies also look a little ridiculous trying to walk in them.

- The super-high, stiletto streetwalker look should be contained to the bedroom, if at all.

Choose a classic pump. Classics are timeless and complimentary.

Our insteps and heels, need to make contact with the ground with each step. Our legs look more attractive while w e a r e walking in a classic stiletto pump or a platform pump.

A classic heeled shoe worked wonders for Marilyn Monroe in the film "Niagara." The scene, in which she walks far away, was one continuous shot, with no cuts, showing her womanly walk. After the release of the film, the sales of high heels skyrocketed.

Robert Palmer lamented about being "Addicted to Love" in his music video, surrounded by stillettoed supermodels. None of them needed Frankenstein shoes to look sexy. Just sayin'.

27. A variety of sexy shoes

One way for me to tell you if you have turned into "Sweat Pants and Baseball Cap" lady is if I were to go into your closet right now and inspect your high-heeled shoe selection. Have you turned sensible in your shoe wardrobe? Now, I'm not saying that we don't need to have comfy stand-on-our-feet or shop-all-day shoes. I have had to invest in a wardrobe of not very attractive squishy padded shoes so I can stand and do hair all day, and not-too-sexy low-heeled breathable boots for on-set wear.

But for all else, do you have a selection of provocative shoes that show your sexy side? It's Not Over Yet! You still want to have the **Beauty Power** to create that illusion of streamlined, sexy elegance.

We know that high heels are a tool to help you look as hot as possible, but do you know that high heels also improve your posture, elongate your form and push the breasts forward? Just slipping them on adjusts your mind-set about your womanliness. Am I right on this? Yes!

Sally Do list of your "It's Not Over Yet!" shoe wardrobe:

- Neutral-toned heel with invisible platform (taupe or tan)

- Black patent leather high heel

- Red stiletto or sling back (strap in the back)

- Bronze, gold or silver slip on mule (i.e.: Betty Grable or classic 1950s Barbie shoe)

If you are having foot/leg/hip issues and simply cannot wear the sex goddess footwear, check out brands like Bjorn, Sofft and The Walking Company. They feature styles that have an edge but are comfy too.

28. Opaque black hose

A fashion staple that never goes out of vogue, and gives a long, leaner look, is the wearing of opaque black hose, paired with a simple black dress. Add some cute platform boots and you will rock the 1960s supermodel vibe. This look works especially well for those of us who have great shaped legs but may not want to bare it all in a slightly shorter dress or skirt. Perhaps you are concerned about leg issues (I'm not going to go into them here, but you know what I mean). You still want to wear dresses and show some leg after 40. Opaque hose are a great way to wear a shorter skirt, feel sexy and hip, and remain age- appropriate.

29. Botox

I admit it. I had my first Botox experience just this past year. I was one of those anti-Botox people. I just couldn't get behind walking around with that surprised look all the time but, just as with the positive hair extension examples, I had to be led to it by seeing others with natural looking results. It has been a whole year since I had the "11's" area, (The furrows between the eyebrows that form a number 11) injected with a small amount. The deep furrow I had there is not glaring anymore. I just look more rested. And no, I did not go on a binge and start Botoxing my entire face, but some people do, and that is unfortunate. Moderation is the key here more than ever. Always go conservative and understated. Overkill can put a person into the "What happened to her?" zone very easily.

Sally's Botox Beauty Rule #1: Get a referral from a friend who is happy with the results. DO NOT pick someone from an ad or go for the DEAL. This is one of those don't-go-cheap absolutes!

Sally's Botox Beauty Rule #2: Go minimal and in only one area, no matter how much the facility may try to up sell you. Once you have lived with it for a while, you can try a second area or move into a filler product for nasolabial folds, etc. for other areas on your face. Here again, please go slowly and gingerly. I would rather keep that wrinkle or soft jowl than walk around looking like "The joker."

Many people are simply not informed about what Botox really is. It's a purified protein that is administered through tiny injections between the brows, to reduce the signs of aging. It works by blocking nerve impulses, which stops the movement of those muscles. With less movement, the skin surface gradually smooths out, and your frown lines begin to fade. Over time, the Botox weakens and dissipates, and everything goes back to the way it was. The good news here is that Botox is not permanent. Because of my conservative position with anything that can change your features, I like the fact that if it isn't for you, your face goes back to normal in time. I caution you again to choose a top professional on this. My personal artist is Sharon at Etcetera Medi Spa in Santa Clarita, Calif., which is conveniently right next door to my studio!

Botox is not for everyone, but using just a teeny bit worked for me.

30. Blepharoplasty and brow lift

One of the first areas to show aging in the face is around the eyes. Fine lines around the eyes slowly make their appearance, and the eyelids begin to droop and lose elasticity, giving a permanent tired look to the entire face. Blepharoplasty, combined with an endoscopic eyebrow lift, is a simple surgical cosmetic procedure that can take 10 years off the face, when done conservatively.

Earlier I shared my mama's cosmetic surgery advice. I really did go to see three doctors and get three consultations, although I already knew who I was going with. It is your FACE, for goodness sakes! I wanted to be 100 percent certain that the RIGHT person was going to slice into my face! I also wanted to know that I would be listened to, and validated, about how I wanted it done. You must go to a doctor you feel comfortable with.

Do your research:

Find out if your chosen doctor is board certified. If not, keep looking. How many of these particular surgeries has he/she done? Are you seeing examples of his/her actual work, or stock photos, a standard library of pictures used in marketing materials and on websites?

Don't be intimidated into having an additional procedure done unless it is truly warranted. This is another example of being up-sold. Be careful not to let this happen. It's like going into an auto dealership and falling for the shiny red sports car, when your plan that morning was to drive away in a nice, practical, affordable model.

I believe in a conservative approach to all procedures. When I went in for a blepharoplasty (eyelid surgery) consultation, my doctor explained that adding an endoscopic (no scalpel or major cutting) brow lift would make the overall look more successful, and make the results last longer, based on my age and rate of facial aging, In this case, I saw that doing an additional procedure was the right choice for me.

An endoscopic brow lift is done by making two small incisions on the forehead; the skin is pulled up slightly. The incisions are in the hairline and are completely undetectable.

A full brow lift is done by an incision across the entire hairline. This procedure is more invasive and is intended for those who have a more profound skin slackening.

It has been eight years, and I'm still looking pretty good in that area. I am happy I did this one thing for myself. I took the conservative approach and I'm glad I did.

For some women, getting only their eyes done will not be enough. If the facial skin is heavily wrinkled, a laser resurfacing or facelift procedure should be considered.

My opinion is that cosmetic procedures should be done earlier rather than later, depending on your rate of aging.

In most cases, a small amount of Botox and some filler (Restalyne or Juvaderm) can keep you looking great for several years.

Fillers are liquid substances that are derived from hyaluronic acid (bovine) that are liquefied, injected into the body and settle into a gel. After about six months or so, the injected substance is absorbed by the body.

As of this writing, I have not had the experience of fillers. I have heard from some ladies who are very satisfied and from some who said they didn't see enough difference to warrant spending the money. It is something that you will have to test out for yourself.

I eventually will try it, so I will have to let you know my experience in my next book. ☺

Further, a simple chin tightening can do wonders for your profile. If I decide to do any additional corrections as I mature, I will look into this option. This will mean an actual surgery and, in addition to having adjustments on sagging eyelids, I believe sharpening the jawline is the best aesthetic improvement we can do, without going into a face-lift.

Thermage is a procedure you may consider; it can firm up the chin area without surgery. This is effective only if you have slight aging in the jawline. If you are actually going into the jowl stage, the only way to get effective results is surgery. Sorry!

Take care of your skin now with sunblock, exfoliation, and collagen stimulating creams, and a facelift may be avoided altogether through your 40s and 50s.

31. Photo facials

Photo facial is a generic term for a skin treatment that uses light-based technology. Photo facials have a number of uses but are mostly used for treating brown spots, broken capillaries, and boosting collagen.

The two main types of technology used for photo facials:

LED (light emitting diode) and IPL (intense-pulsed light) are completely different, so it's extremely important to understand which photo facial technology is being used. That way you are more likely to get the results you hope to achieve.

An LED photo facial is a very gentle treatment that uses narrow spectrum light to boost collagen, which creates plumper, younger-looking skin or to kill the bacteria that cause acne. This type of photo facial is likely to be found in a day spa with a serious focus on aesthetics.

LED photo facials are painless, cool and relaxing, and (unlike IPL or laser treatments) carry no risk of burning. The best results come after a series of photo facial treatments. To begin, a series of six treatments with one to two weeks between is recommended. After that, maintain with a treatment every month or two. It can be part of a facial or a stand-alone treatment.

LED photo facials are a good choice for people who want to boost collagen or treat acne. Their collagen-boosting facial rejuvenation properties have been proven with medical research. The results will not be as dramatic as plastic surgery, but it's a gentler, more natural and less expensive way to go.

Some spas call the intense-pulsed light procedure, (IPL), a photo facial. An IPL photo facial can treat a variety of skin conditions such as brown spots, broken capillaries, spider veins and facial redness. An IPL photo facial delivers a bright blast of light at very high energy levels through a hand-held device. Although some IPLs have cooling devices, the treatments can be uncomfortable, even painful.

An IPL photo facial is the better choice if you have brown spots, broken capillaries or overall redness.

The number of IPL photo facials you need will vary depending on the condition you're treating, the results you want and how your skin responds.

The IPL photo facial is the one that I had. I did a series of three and I saw a visible improvement in my rosaceous skin and a slight improvement in my overall sameness of tone.

32. Rainforest lactic peels

I talk about exfoliation a lot. Anyone who really knows the skin will tell you that keeping the surface skin free of dead cells will make it look smoother and more luminescent and allow it to absorb products better. However, the key here is moderation. Some ladies go crazy with the skin peels. Let's think about what our body does naturally to protect itself from invaders and how that process can be slightly assisted to beautify us as well, without harsh, aggressive tactics.

Depending on our age, diet, climate etc., these factors can change a bit, yet any esthetician school student can tell you that our skin naturally turns over every fourteen days. This process is the body's way of pushing the older, drier layers of skin to the surface, allowing the thicker, spongier skin to give needed cover to the body. Thicker skin is bonded more tightly and can better protect the skin from invaders like illness and injury. Our facial skin shows this process when it gets dry and flakey. When our foundation base looks yucky, we start to look tired, dehydrated and, let's be honest here, older than we feel.

If we stay ahead of it and do a light exfoliation once a week, we are assisting the skin in its natural process. That is why I prefer naturally occurring acids like lactic and mixed-fruit acids. I use a lactic acid from the rainforest, along with an orange blossom scrub that is aggressive enough to exfoliate but gentle enough not to irritate. I don't understand why many women still think they need to peel their skin every day and include harsh loofahs in the shower. They think they did a good peel when their faces are red, irritated and scabbed. Anything of that nature should always be done under the supervision of a doctor. Never do any kind of exfoliation that causes blisters, deep redness or scabbing. You could be prematurely aging the skin.

Lactic acids are gentle. When applied to the surface of freshly cleansed skin with a citrus-based scrub, the lactic acid will absorb into the outermost layers and gently loosen any dead cells that are already due to come off. This treatment does not force exfoliation. When I am told I look ten years younger than my actual age, I am certain that these conservative peeling techniques, along with sunscreen, have done their jobs.

I'm going to be a bit unpopular here, but I'm still not convinced that microdermabrasion machines are helping our skin in the long run; I think they are just too aggressive, sandblasting the skin from the top down, again, forcing exfoliation. I'm interested to see what microdermed skin looks like in twenty-five years. The layers of skin that are naturally going to occur in the outermost layers aren't given their chance to surface because they have been forced off from the top, not naturally occurring from the bottom.

33. Dance classes!

Dance to live! Live to dance!

It's amazing how you can get up and go to work one day and not have a clue that you are going to meet someone that particular day who will help you change your perspective and turn you back to the light. This is one of the exciting things about life: waking up every day, wondering what the day has in store.

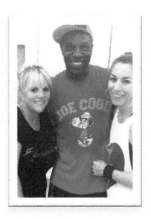

In spring of 2011, I was booked on a Swiffer infomercial with beautiful actress/dancer/Melissa Rivera. I'm always excited to have the opportunity to work with dancers! As the day unfolded, Melissa shared that she danced in the world of popping and locking, a sort of hip-hop style. She jumpstarted her dance career late in the game and was jazzed that at the age of 37 she was a working dancer. We became instant BFFs during the shoot. She mentioned that her boyfriend was an award-winning choreographer. She invited me to take his class. At wrap time, I asked her who he was, and when she told me it was Anthony Thomas, Janet Jackson's Rhythm Nation maestro, I started jumping up and down and gleaming with excitement. It's now been three years that I've been trekking to Anthony's class on Monday nights in North Hollywood, at Debbie Reynolds' famous rehearsal studios, where everyone from Gene Kelly to John Travolta to Justin Bieber have prepped.

Thank you, Melissa, for pushing me to show up. You don't know the huge gift you gave.

Sometimes we need to be nudged a bit just to START something. We want to, but let's be blunt, sometimes we're terrified. I told Melissa I had quit dancing ten years ago and was out of shape, overweight, would never be able keep up, too old, lived too far away, was too busy with daughter, had a business, blah blah blah, but Melissa pressed on, because she sensed the joy I had left behind. It took one class and I was hooked. Anthony's easy-going and passionate teaching style was one I could wrap myself around. This renowned choreographer could just rest on his laurels with what he has already attained in the industry, creating a new style of dance (combining popping and locking), in the 1980s and '90s that would inspire generations of dancers. Anthony is authentically committed to bringing the original street dance style to THIS generation of dancers. Find Anthony Thomas at:

www.anthonythomasdance.com

How AMAZING that I am getting a second chance to be part of the learning experience, just because someone took a minute to include me. I'm actually starting to feel like part of the group now, a great accomplishment. Do I feel awkward, not fit enough, and OLD, compared to the young professionals? Considering that 70% of the class is under 25 and that they travel from all over the world to dance there, I most certainly do, but I deal with it. The fact that I am over 50 and in there DOING IT makes me very proud of myself.

Just do it.

Is there a style of dance you always wanted to try? Just do it, girl. Dancing is one of the most amazing ways to spend an hour or so that I have ever experienced. There are so many types of dance, it's like red lipstick... There is a shade for everyone.

Gyms are featuring **Zumba** classes that will bust you into shape. I think I'm in decent cardio shape for my age, but I struggle hard in a Zumba class. The calorie burning here is at the highest level. If you are trying to take off some pounds, this will do it.

Ballroom dancing is great for a non-dancer and one of the best ways to reconnect with your honey, if you can get him there. You may be pleasantly surprised to find he loves it even more than you do! Once connected to it, men love the feeling of being able to lead the woman; it is very romantic. Encourage him to at least try it. It will be something you can do together to keep the connection.

Tap dancing is a major calorie burner and just plain fun! Do you want sexy, strong legs into your 80s? Tap it. In Palm Springs there is a group of ladies ages 50 to 80 who perform "The Follies." Checking that out and seeing the shape these ladies are in will get you to enroll in tap dancing classes immediately!

Lyrical jazz (my favorite dance style) takes years to perfect but that's what makes it so enjoyable: You find yourself getting better and stronger every week. But let me warn you, it is addicting, so watch out! If you are in Los Angeles, check out Millennium, Debbie Reynolds and Edge Dance Studios.

By the way, if you try a class or two and it doesn't seem quite right for you, it may be your instructor. Not every teacher's style is the best for YOU. I have taken classes from some talented choreographers whom I just could NOT follow, and others I stayed with for YEARS. Find the right teacher and you will find the right fit.

Michael Rooney, son of dancer/actor Mickey Rooney, was the perfect teacher for me through the 1990s for lyrical jazz. He was fun, focused on technique with repetition to execute learning and, most important, validated my improvement. Some instructors can be drill sergeants and taskmasters, with a tough love teaching style. That might work for you, or maybe not. Find which way of teaching matches your learning style.

Dance reshapes your body in a way that no other exercise does; it elongates your body, improves your posture and focuses your brain. The discipline it requires eventually reveals a true passion, when your body performs a movement that you have trained it to do. Such a sense of accomplishment!

I believe dance is so much more rewarding than just going to the gym.

This is especially great for a body that is starting to show and feel its age. I think dancing creates reverse aging! I challenge you to try some form of dance for six months. See what it does not only to your body but for your attitude!

Dance gives you an edge and brings back a little bit of your youth.

34. Hiking/Walking

When I was younger, hiking was just boring. Tromping through the mountains or walking for hours just left me antsy. I went on these little excursions once in a while with my friends or family just to go along with the program, but after the birth of my daughter and the weight gain that came with it, I heard that walking was the tried and true way to keep it off permanently. I tried going on the treadmill at the gym and running and I REALLY hated that. So I gave walking and hiking another try and found it to be enlightening.

What I learned is that long walks can clear your head. You can solve some of your life dilemmas while walking or hiking and being In the moment with yourself. I've come up with my best ideas while on hikes! Buddy it up sometimes too, because while you are walking and talking, it's amazing how time goes by so quickly, and before you know it you are done! **Walking and hiking keep your legs toned and muscular.** By our 50s, the skin around the knees and the upper thighs begins to get jelly-ish. Yuck! We must fight this off as long as possible. Hiking at an incline, up a mountain, rewards you with the results of a Stairmaster and is much more soulful. Girls, if you say to me here, "but I hate hiking!" then as a last resort, grab your iPod and just set a goal to walk for 20 minutes. DO IT!

35. Yoga

The same week that I enrolled in hair school, back in 2003, my sister started going to yoga. I've watched yoga transform her body to give her an improved posture, strong shoulders and a shapelier butt. She is committed to her yoga practice and it has paid off.

I really HATE yoga. I'm too hyper for that type of thing. I hate the down dogs and the planks; they're just downright uncomfortable. I'm in class thinking what is wrong with all these people! This is torture! I am so out of here! BUT I make myself stay, and the results DO pay off.

I sleep better. I'm mellower. My tummy loses the bloat. My arms feel and look leaner, tauter. I am forced to be in the moment with myself. Some people love yoga from their first class. For me, it's a process. I'm still working on it, but I know that I MUST continue with the practice, because yoga teaches us to just slow down and breathe, and as we are maturing, yoga is channeling our bodies to strength and power. **Beauty Power!**

36. Music

It's simple. Load your favorite tunes of all time on to your iPod and ENJOY. Little did we know, way back then, that one day we could program our favorite tunes into one spot! Technology rocks!

What about going out to enjoy your favorite music in an atmosphere that relaxes you? Investigate where they are playing the stuff that feeds your inner joy. Go listen!

Remember the awesome rocked-out concerts in your teens and 20s? Google your favorite band. Is it coming to town? Just go rock out.

37. Radiance through nutrition

I'm not in a position to give nutritional advice, but I have made some permanent lifestyle changes I would like to share.

Through my adult years, my sugar addiction kept me from being at my best and kept me from slimming down as curvy/lean as I would prefer to be, compared to too curvy! I generally ate healthful food, but I ate too much of it (it's the American way!). I am learning to eat smaller amounts of carbs like bread and potatoes while adding larger portions of salad and veggies to my plate, so I won't feel cheated.

These past few years I trimmed 20 pounds and have kept it off. There is more to go, but my doctor is proud that I have made some permanent lifestyle changes. Luckily, I discovered early the benefits of tomatoes, salmon, fiber, pineapple, sweet potatoes and lean protein, like turkey.

Some of the foods I CURRENTLY include in my diet for energy, digestion and skin radiance:

Salmon, turkey, pineapple, kale, avocado, almonds, broccoli, edamame, almond milk, coconut milk, raw cranberry juice, lemons, Ezekiel bread (flourless), red wine, dark chocolate and an occasional steak.

I AVOID greasy foods (OK, French fries are an exception!), anything breaded or deep fried, pork sausage, pork bacon, sandwich meats (with the exception of sliced lean turkey breast), most red meats and most fast food. Cookies are my weakness. I find most of the time I have to try tojust avoid them all together. It's sad that I can't control myself once a platter of cookies is presented. But you know girls, It's Not Over Yet!. We MUST treat ourselves sometimes. When I am working on set, craft services will present some ridiculously yummy dessert and cookies to die for! Arggh! I beeline over, grab one or two and then avoid that area for the rest of the shoot. If you too are a sugar junkie, search out LOTS of good placebo desserts to satisfy you most of the time and treat yourself to something decadent and wonderful some of the time. That's what has worked for me. My favorites are Weight Watchers

Tres Leches frozen bars and Skinny Cow Caramel Truffle bars. 100 calories.

Ladies, water is an ABSOLUTE must in our second half, to keep our digestive systems working and our skin plumped! Another big challenge for me: drinking enough water. Recently I discovered that drinking bottled water at room temperature helps me get MORE WATER into my body daily. Try it.

A model gave me a GREAT tip once about dining out and not overdoing it. She decides in advance if she is going to have wine, bread OR dessert, but only one of the three. I try to do that one. It doesn't always work, but at least it's in my head.

What I'm going to do in my second half? Enjoy good, yummy, healthful food AND keep my **Beauty Power!**

38. Sexuality and intimacy—Get your playful on

Not long ago, I was working on set with a gorgeous blonde actress. She had some acne on her skin that I was concealing. Her acne was her beauty hang-up, the thing that kept her from flawlessness.

We got into a deep discussion about how we wonder about what a lover is thinking during intimate times, when we might obsess about our breasts and our bellies.

This stunning, playful beauty and I entertained ourselves with jokes about it, even though there was truth behind our laughter. Then she said something that I will take with me forever. "Most men aren't thinking about of ANY of that. They're just happy to be there!"

Ladies, if you get this one thing from my book, the rest can be a fun read, because you have gotten the message.

The #1 issue many men have with their partners is the lack of attention. It's not your ten extra pounds, the lines on your face or the burnt dinner. Most men aren't focused on those things. They want to be loved in bed, kissed in the morning and, most important, to be validated!

They want to know that you SEE them and what they are trying to do for you and the family. This goes back to the Stone Age days, when men wereconditioned to be providers. They were the hunters and the gatherers. We women were the nurturers. This ingrained behavior carries over to present day, when men still take on the responsibility, even if they are not the sole providers; it's still in their DNA.

A little unconditional sex goes a long way to make your man happy and keep the relationship healthy. You don't feel like it. I don't blame you. Sometimes I have come home to a family that has been waiting for the night to start. It's on pause until I come in. "Mommy's home. What's for dinner?" OMG. Are you kidding me?? I've been standing on my feet all day! I'm tired!

Then after dinner and dishes, we are supposed to be hot lovers? Forget this. I'm going to check OUT.

Does this scenario sound familiar? We have to remember, what about our man? Did he also work his twelve hours? All he really wants is some validation and affection.

As George Carlin said, "All men really want is (fill in the blank) and a sandwich." We have to remember that they are men and they are different than we are. We can't expect them to respond to the same triggers we do. Men are men. MEN are NOT like us!

Life Lesson: *Men like to make little sexual innuendos and tap you on the butt, etc. I used to REALLY be annoyed by this. I would react negatively to this kind of attention. But the truth is that they are just trying to connect. It's their attempt to get some kind of reaction. Pay attention to this behavior from your partner. It's OK to tell him you don't feel comfortable with this approach, but say it with the kindest of words. Let him know you welcome his advances, but perhaps they can happen in a different manner. The main thing is communication. If we don't like the way something is being done or said, put it into words.*

If we continue to shut down our man every time he approaches, one day he may give up and just stop. Then we wonder why he is not loving us. He still loves us; he is just not "loving" us anymore. This is the dangerous time when he may be starting to notice other women, even though in most cases he won't do anything. But slowly, the eroding of the relationship begins, and one day we wonder where it went. We just cannot blame ALL of our relationship issues on him.

It doesn't diminish us to laugh at little jokes we may think are not funny or to be playful even when we are not quite there. And it is OK to tell a man "not tonight honey" because we just can't get into the sexual mood. However, if we promise that tomorrow night will be different, let's find a way to amp up our brain and make sure it happens. He will spend that entire day thinking about what's going to happen. If we rebuff him again, then it might create more hostility. Don't make empty promises.

It is amazing to me how men respond to a woman's attention. We worry that some younger, hotter chick will lead him away, yet in most cases men leave for women who are not even as attractive as their wives. It is the woman who gives him attention and listens to him that you need to be most concerned about. You know this, girls, and I am reminding you. Trust me, I know it because I have lived it and do not plan to make that mistake in my second half.

Some relationships have it the other way around. This is particularly maddening for us over-40 ladies whose bodies aren't as rock solid as before babies, age and stress. Your man has become contented in the relationship, is a bit bored and has stopped making love to you. What used to be hours doing it on your living room floor has become once a month. DO NOT go with the flow on this one, ladies. Communicate!! Don't assume it's your less-than-perky boobs or your little jelly belly. As I said before, it is usually NOT THAT, unless you picked a guy who is shallow, and that's a problem you should have addressed when you noticed him checking out other women on the first date. Next!

Perhaps his long hours and stress on the job, combined with your own exhaustion, have made it easier to let it slide. He is getting older too, and things aren't working as quickly as when he was 30. As we age and our workload increases, it is natural to want to settle at the end of the day into a cozy routine of kicking back and watching a movie, grabbing a yummy dessert and watching other people live their lives on reality shows or following the weekly story line of "Mad Men," just to decompress our brains.

This is bad-bad! Watching TV doesn't make us want our men. It makes us sedentary, as we compare our lives to fantasy lives we imagine. It makes us discontented with our mates, because they are not anything like the current hottie. WE get compared to 18–year-old, 6-foot, 100-pound Victoria's Secret models who are blasted on commercials and print ads.

Hey! I have an idea. Power down! Turn the TV OFF!

My mom used to call the TV the idiot box. I'm beginning to see her point.

It's OK to have NO TV a couple of nights a week. Find something that HE is interested in doing and do it with him! Dirt bike riding would not be #1 on my list of interests, yet when my family began going on regular trips to the desert, I decided it was way better to be with them than without. I learned to ride a quad dirt bike and enjoy weekends in the desert. It turned out to be fun, and it connected us as a family.

After a couple of trips of my Gosh-I-hate-this attitude, something unexpected happened. I actually started to LIKE it, because I got better at it. Is it just because it's not your idea that you don't want to try something new? Pick one thing your husband/boyfriend is into and just TRY it.

What has your husband/boyfriend asked you to do with him that so far you have not tried?

What about something NEW that you can try together? I'm learning how to golf. A year ago I would have laughed off the idea and told you golf is for old people. However, I drive by a golf course many days. I noticed the people who play golf look fit and relaxed. Every golfer I have ever met has a mellow vibe and is usually successful. That sounds good to me. I'm at least checking it out. If it's not for me I will stay with my dancing, but how do you know about anything that you have never tried yourself?

I see a lot of post-40 women pulling away and disconnecting from their partners.

I hear ladies talking about hot actors and sports stars they crush on. I don't really get this. Because I work in the entertainment and sports industries, I often have the opportunity to work with the real people whom we, in a media frenzied society, have built up into megastars. I see them standing there or sitting in my makeup chair, looking like more stylized and fit versions of ourselves. They are just people doing their jobs, as we are doing ours.

A Sally Aha! Moment. I'm not much for the star-struck experience, but there was one A List film and TV actor whom I had a little crush on for years. To my joy, he appeared on our call sheet one spring morning when we were setting up to do public service promotions for NBC's "The More You Know."

The lead makeup artist knew I had a "thing," so when he arrived in the makeup room, she generously directed him to my chair and watched for the show to begin. Ha ha.

As my celebrity crush approached my makeup station with that camera-ready- sexy smile, I sheepishly shook his hand for several seconds, smiling an embarrassing goober smile, until the seconds became uncomfortably long. I had watched this actor for several years in films and on TV and envisioned him as he was usually cast; the ruggedly handsome boyfriend with a sensitive side.

In my chair, he was friendly, talkative, kind, engaging, yet slightly aloof. However, when he stood next to me, I couldn't get over how small and lean he was in person. He was only slightly taller than I, and although definitely cute, he didn't look like he could actually kick much ass. Wow. That was a little bit of letdown.

This is it. I realized that day that I had purchased the fantasy but that in real life, he was just a handsome guy who had beat hundreds of hopeful actors to get a part and had built that part into a career and had became famous. He was making a lucrative living out of being our fantasy man, the guy-next-door type we wish we could meet. Ladies, don't waste years on the fantasy train, wishing your guy could be someone else. Enjoy the living, breathing one you have in front of you. Right now put this book down and, if you have a husband or boyfriend, go to him and give him a slow tender kiss.

You can finish reading this book tomorrow.

39. Attitude adjustment

I think at some point we just have to make a decision. Getting older really sucks, and no woman is thrilled about it, but think of the alternative. There are so many fabulous things about maturing, I could go on forever.

Think about how smart we are, what we have learned through life lessons and what we want in relationships NOW, in this second half, think about what we can do with those lessons. Think about how we can help and guide others.

Think about how we can finally start to plan for that trip to Paris that we have always dreamed of. In California, the Automobile Club has a plan for people who dream that one day they will go somewhere. Through a special travel savings package, they can book a tour and pay it off in monthly payments for two years. Go ahead, girl. Book your trip to Europe now!

This year I am going to Memphis to see Graceland. Always wanted to see it but just haven't taken the time to make the trip. I want to take my daughter to Chicago for the holidays; I'll do that too.

Where do YOU want to go?

One of the saddest stories I heard in my adult years was something my sweet brother Geoff told me about our dad. Our real father, an award-winning landscape designer, did many exciting things in his lifetime, and he always dreamed of seeing Africa. He talked about it for years but just never made it there. That is NOT happening to me because I am going to plan for the trip and make it.

Getting back to dance was something I put off for 10 years, but I DID go back.

What have you put off doing that you daydream about?

What trip do you want to take that you are still talking about?

How much time do you think you really have?

Stephanie the Gladiator

My sister Stephanie thought she had run out of time. She had noticed a large lump inside the front of her tummy. She asked me to feel it to see if I felt anything strange. I was a nurse's aide in my late teens, so my family considered that the closest thing to a nurse!

I applied pressure on the upper abdomen and I immediately noticed a prominent round lump, like a small orange. I tried to act calm but I was alarmed. Like many ladies who take care of others first, she had previously shrugged it off. She had

---

noticed this lump weeks earlier but thought it could be a hernia, or perhaps she was just bloated!

Her doctor discovered that she had stage 3 ovarian cancer, and it was moving quickly. So just as quickly, Stephanie fought like a gladiator and took control. With her daughter Laurel, my niece, at her side every step of the way, she had major surgery, a hysterectomy, and a 10- pound malignant tumor was removed successfully. Then on to rounds of chemo, successful because she strictly and steadfastly followed orders from her doctor and the staff at City of Hope.

Stephanie, at 72, is cancer-free. Her oncologist shared with her that he watched a 40-year-old patient with the same diagnosis die. He didn't understand it medically, because she had been given the same treatment. The difference here was Stephanie's unfailingly POSITIVE attitude, disarming everyone around her.

We all had begun to accept that this cancer would kill her, but Stephie was NOT going to have it. She was going to take that first step and face her fear. I named her Gladiator. She loved that name, and it was so fitting a description of the way she carried herself through this journey.

Stephanie doesn't take anything for granted. Her amazing ATTITUDE will take her through the next part of her life. She celebrated her new life in Ireland and continues to plan and make trips.

I'm not saying that I believe a great attitude will cure your cancer. I'm saying that a POSITIVE, forward-moving attitude is one of the most powerful gifts that only YOU can give yourself.

NO ONE CAN GIVE IT OR TAKE IT FROM YOU. Stephanie taught me, and I am sure many others, this life lesson. Attitude adjustment is a choice.

Despite your current typecast, you can always choose a different role.

If you are not in love with who you are, fall in love with who you can become.

IT'S NOT OVER YET!

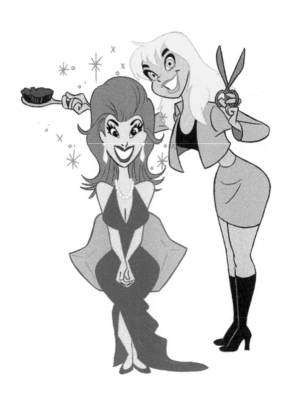

CHAPTER 5

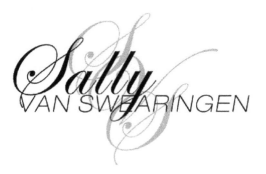
Sally
VAN SWEARINGEN

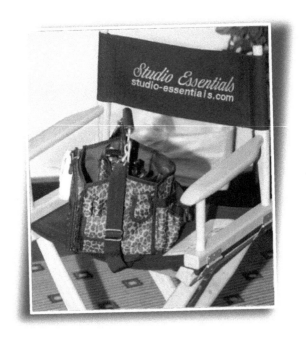

Insert celebrity (or you!) here.

Celebrity and High-Profile Interactions: What the Stars Taught Me

- Star Gazing

- Being "In the Moment"

- Role Models

- In Transition

When I began this book, my book coach Judith strongly suggested that I include some of the stories of my celebrity interactions. She had heard several of them and was convinced that my desired audience would want to hear these stories too. I initially doubted that my readers would be interested in these little life lessons, but Judith pressed on.

I began to explore in my mind the many on-set places I have gone and the fascinating people from whom I have been lucky enough to have learned nuggets of wisdom. Of the special people I write about here, some were experiencing stardom on the rise, and some were transitioning to the other side, in different stages of their lives and different stages of mine. I realized there is a story here.

Star Gazing

Gene Kelly: Dancer, Singer, Actor

Although I never did meet Gene Kelly, there are two lessons here.

Gene Kelly made a statement on the Johnny Carson show in the 1970s, that inspired me, and I never, ever forgot. Johnny was flattering him about his talent as a dancer. Gene Kelly talked about how you can be the most talented and well-trained dancer on the planet; there are thousands of them. Training and discipline is important, yes. Luck is important, yes. But the most important thing to achieve great success in anything you aspire to be is sheer determination. Determination is what will eventually get you there.

At 17, I was moving to Alabama with my parents. The week before we moved, my friends and I shared all the things we would do if we were forced to leave California. Mine:

1. See Grauman's Chinese Theatre.

2. Meet Gene Kelly.

My Chatsworth High School dancer friends and I spent a glorious day and evening truly discovering Hollywood as never before, spending hours on Hollywood Boulevard and at Grauman's, checking out the famous footprints of Marilyn Monroe, Bette Davis and all of our favorites. We scooted over to Famous Amos cookies on Sunset and La Brea (Wally Amos had a store there until he became a global brand) and the Max Factor museum. My dancer friend Lori was a Liza Minnelli fanatic, knew her family and had an inside track on knowing where the stars lived.

Gene Kelly lived on Canon Drive in Beverly Hills. It was decided that we were going there to meet him! This was the mid 1970s, when things were a little mellower and a person could actually walk up to a door and attempt to meet their star.

We arrived at the Kelly house, which was modest by Beverly Hills standards. With gentle prodding, the girls convinced me to go up to the front door and ring the bell. I clutched the famous glossy of him caressing a street banister in "Singing in the Rain,", holding it close to my chest. I rang the doorbell. An eternity of seconds. Then a woman, talking through the closed door and slightly annoyed, asked if she could help me. In an overly sweet tone, I answered back. "Oh, YES, you certainly can! I'm Sally. I am a dancer too, and I am here to meet Mr. Kelly and have him sign my photograph of him. I'm moving to Alabama next week and this is my last chance to meet him!"

Another eternity of seconds. "Slip it under the door, please, with your name and address. Mr. Kelly is in New York and he will be there for several weeks. Thank You." I was like "huh?" I don't get to meet Gene Kelly?" And why should I leave the picture? They won't send it to me. After taking it all in and accepting my fate, I turned and walk away, dejected.

Life lesson learned?

In the years since, I have slapped myself a hundred times. Why Sally, did you NOT leave the picture, which cost you $3? I'm sure they probably would have mailed the autographed Gene Kelly picture. Duh.

We have all had these experiences, but now we know that we probably will not get a second chance. Do it NOW. What are we afraid of? These are the types of experiences that we simply just won't have again in our second half, because we have learned better.

Chuck Berry: Singer, Songwriter

I'm 19 and at the Denny's Coffee Shop on Century Boulevard near LAX Airport. Sitting in the coffee shop a few booths from ours is singer-songwriter-musician-icon, Chuck Berry. He is smoking a cigarette and drinking black coffee. His recent resurgence in the media through B-roll concert footage included in "American Graffiti" and other musicals made him easy for this blues lover to spot.

I had much more chutzpah in those days, that is for sure. With zero hesitation, I approach him immediately. "Uh, hi. Excuse me, are you Chuck

Berry?" The relaxed, slightly distracted grin told me that he was pleased to be recognized.

"Yeah, it's me darlin'." His grayish/black skin was deeply lined, telling a story of intense traveling, late nights and hard partying. How I would have loved to have been invited to sit and just listen. I was thinking of "Back in the U.S.A.," "Maybellene" and the many stories to be told around it. But with all the fame, this man sat there totally Zen, taking a breather from it all.

Many people passed; very few noticed him. I was shocked!. My moment with Chuck Berry told me of a man who appreciated his fame and the money that enabled him to play music, but at the end of the day, with all of his infamy, here was a man enjoying another day of life, relaxing with a cigarette and cup of joe. Damn, that was a special moment.

Shirley Jones: Singer, Actress

This is one of my most embarrassing and "omigosh! Where is a hole to fall in to?" moments. At 21, my first paid job as makeup artist was working at the Long Beach Civic light Opera, as a makeup assistant. My job was to do the décolleté (chest) makeup on the performers. Basically, I powdered their chests and painted shadows between their breasts to create cleavage. One of my duties was to stand offstage near the curtain to apply last-minute powder as the busty ladies entered the stage. Shirley Jones was the star of this turn of the century musical, "Bittersweet."

The costumes, as with many stage and opera shows, were ornate, full, and heavy.

One night I was standing in my usual spot, holding my tools, but this night I guess I had my foot sticking out. Before I could see or hear (because I am hearing-impaired and have been known to get distracted), Shirley Jones came fluttering by me in a haste, rushing to the stage for what was obviously a late curtain call. Ker-plump! She was down. "Oh no! I tripped the star of the show!"

Without a beat and with the skill of an Olympic athlete, Miss Jones rose to her feet, glided onto the stage and met her cue to perfection.

I will never forget my shock, both at what I had done and at the agility and quick reflexes of a lifelong film and stage performer. Shirley Jones was in her 50s at the time, but the adrenaline effect worked its magic, and all was wonderful in the world. I slowly sank back from the shadowy curtain and tried to disappear. I just knew I was going to be canned that night. My career in the opera would be short and sweet. But something amazing happened. Nobody talked about it, no one mentioned it. Should I say something? I wretched and wretched. That night I asked my stepdad, who was, as far as I was concerned, Moses on the mountain in giving advice. After a few moments of thought, he came up with this: "Will there be any time that you will be in the company of Shirley Jones privately?"

"Well, probably not. When I powder her breasts, the makeup designer is always with me, doing her face." He advised that if no one is saying anything, I should leave it alone unless I got a chance to talk to her alone.

The wrap party for "Bittersweet" was held at the home of Shirley Jones and husband, Marty Engels. I decided to throw myself on my sword and tell her. I really had to get this off my chest! Somehow I got the courage to start a conversation.. She thanked me for my fine breast building skills and we smiled. Then I hit her with it.

"Um, Miss Jones. Um. I was the one who tripped you that night. I didn't mean to." She looked a little confused, with a raised eyebrow. Then, connecting to the moment, she began to laugh, really laugh. Marty offered a slight disapproving look for a second, and then he began to laugh too. They giggled in unison, perhaps at my expense for getting up the nerve to admit my blunder when it was so NOT a big deal. At that point, I realized that they both were feeling good from the wine. Marty began to play the piano, and I was off the hook.

I realized right then that getting up after a fall was the core to longevity in the entertainment business and perhaps in life. No matter who or what trips you, just dust yourself off and get up.

Thank you, Shirley Jones, for an amazing life lesson that I have carried with me for over Thirty years!

Being "In the Moment"

Being in the moment was Michael Landon's philosophy.

Although I never had the pleasure of meeting the much admired actor-producer-director-role model Michael Landon, who died way too soon after a much publicized, brave fight with pancreatic cancer, I did have the pleasure of working with a close friend of his, blind actor-activist-entrepreneur Tom Sullivan, who shared with me that Michael Landon's example in life was being "in the moment" with whomever he was with; focusing all of his attention on that person.

Michael advised him early in his career to always take the time to be in the moment are with someone. The person you are with will be honored by this. Since this was shared with me, I have aspired to always be in the moment, although it's one of the most challenging things a person can do.

Here are some glimpses into those moments:

Dolly Parton: Singer, Songwriter, Entrepreneur

We hear stories of mega celebrities who took time out of their day to do something magical for a fan. It actually did happen to me and was one of the early driving forces of my success in life.

In 1982 I was 25 years old. I was loving life because I had secured a coveted spot as a tour guide at Universal Studios. To ace the audition, I told a funny Dolly Parton story.

A couple of months and about 50 tram tours later, I heard that Dolly would be filming "The Best Little Whorehouse in Texas" on the lower lot.

By this time, it had become common knowledge to the other tour guides that I LOVED Dolly. Dolly stories were my favorite stall material when the trams got backed up. Word spread throughout the lot that I was a fan. Many people tried to arrange a meeting with Dolly, and a couple of times it got close. When summer came around, I auditioned to work for the special effects stages, mainly because I knew SHE was filming down there and that would give me a better chance to get on the set. Months passed, and the opportunity did not present itself, even though we tried.

One sad summer day it was announced that Dolly had wrapped filming. She was going back to Tennessee. I was disappointed that my one opportunity to meet her had passed: so close and yet so far away. Dolly Parton was becoming a MEGASTAR. Her face and body glazed all the major magazines. The National Enquirer, Star Magazine, and Johnny Carson chose Dolly as one of their favorites to mock. For a rising star, that's the best P.R. you can get!

Now I would never meet her and never be allowed the opportunity to get to her. Wah!

But, It's Not Over Yet!.

Forward to December 1982. One of my tour guide friends, an actor, called me at home to say Dolly was again on the lot, filming pick up shots for a musical number. They had built an entire four-wall façade inside the soundstage, where they could film Dolly from all angles, exiting a staircase for her number. Shooting would take only a couple of days, I was told. So my friend Jennifer, a cute blonde actress with an ingenious plan, decided that we were going to use our Universal IDs to gain entrance to the lot and get inside Stage 24, the largest soundstage, where Dolly was doing her thing.

It was a rainy day that December. I lugged along a huge framed lithograph of Dolly playing a guitar that my parents had given me a few years earlier, trying hard not to get it wet. Maybe I would be lucky enough to meet her and at least have her sign it. Isn't it interesting how when something major happens in our lives, we remember what we were wearing, what song was playing. I remember exactly what I was wearing that day. I hadn't yet discovered my **Beauty Power** or what my personal style would be. My ensemble was a burgundy brown corduroy skirt, paired with a fancy silk blouse tied high at the neck and pink cowboy boots! What can I say? At the time, I thought Dolly would like it.

Somehow Jennifer and I got on the lot with the expired tour guide IDs, although we were no longer working there! WE even made our way into the sound stage. We were pretty, 25-year-old blondes then, so I'm sure that helped.

We schmoozed our way onto the secured stage. Jennifer did most of the talking and I just smiled. She told them that Dolly was expecting us because she was going to sign the picture, which she had forgotten to do months before, after meeting us on the tour (as if Dolly took the tour??). The made-up story sounded real good to me, and I just kept smiling.

Now we were on the lot and on the set. Getting to Dolly was the question. After waiting on the sidelines, sitting on a bench for the longest time, we were finally guided to a more comfortable observation spot and invited to watch filming. We sat and enjoyed watching several takes of Dolly covering the soundtrack as she descended the stairs, in her beaded, skin-tight red dress.

After the final take, Dolly was escorted back to her huge bus. As she brushed past us, all I could come up with was "Hi." She tossed me that Dolly laugh and said, "Well, how are ya?" She was breathtakingly beautiful. This was years before I worked with or touched the face of anyone famous, and Dolly was one of the biggest rising stars of that moment in time.

I was completely star-struck. It was the one and only time I truly ever was, but I will never forget it.

Within seconds she was past me and clicking up the steps in her stiletto heels, to enter her mansion on wheels, the same bus that Barbara Walters had shown to millions on national TV. I sat dumbfounded, holding my huge glass lithograph.

The security guard, God bless him, scooted up to her and offered that we had been there ALL day, waiting to meet her. Dolly glanced over at her eager young fan and quickly became involved in the scenario. "Well, come on in!" were her first words to me, in that beautiful giggly, Southern tone that a person doesn't forget. Jennifer nudged me to go on ahead and, of course, I did.

I climbed the steps into the bus, and it was truly glamorous. Dolly smiled at me with the warmest smile. She said something to me about waiting here a minute while she changed and I was dazed. "Is this a dream? Am I really here?" Seconds later, she reappeared in another gorgeous dress, but I couldn't tell you the color. I only remember her milky white, translucent skin and sculpted, high cheekbones. Although voluptuous, she was a tiny lady who came up to my nose and seemed half my size. Her beauty transcended anything that I could have imagined, and I remember thinking "Wow. THIS is what a movie star looks like up close."

Dolly was concerned about the lithograph solidly pressed into the frame, behind the glass, and how we were going to retrieve it. She sat there, in her gorgeous gown, on her glamour bus couch and attempted to take it out with her exquisitely manicured long nails!!! This worried me right away. OH, NO! Would she break a nail for me? Man, I am in trouble.

Happily, she soon determined that this was a job for professionals. She summoned the security guard and asked if he could grab one of the prop guys to get it out. While waiting for the return of the picture, I was given an amazing few minutes with Dolly, in the moment. Dolly was gifting me with precious movie-making time. Real time. Everything stopped. She asked about my career. I babbled about my facial work and making brides look pretty. I'm sure whatever I said wasn't making sense, but she got the gist.

She said that she would have been a beautician if the music thing hadn't worked out.

(We all saw Dolly's actual hairdressing skills in the film "Steel Magnolias," in which she played a beauty shop owner) She told me to always believe in myself and said I could do whatever I wanted in life. Last, she told me not to worry about other people and what they think. I wish I had taken that third bit of Dolly wisdom with me through life, but I know for a fact the first two Dolly gems became part of me.

Dolly Parton did the one thing with me that later huge successes have also done. She was in the moment for that brief space in time and, in being so, helped me secure the decision of where I was going in my chosen profession.

Dolly Parton became an even bigger movie and musical star, songwriter, author, producer, theme park creator, you name it, and she remains one of the most successful entrepreneurs in the country.

I believe Dolly and I will meet again someday.

Danny Bonaduce: Actor

Danny Bonaduce is one of the most down-to-earth, REAL actor-entertainers that I have had the pleasure to work with. I learned a lot from him by observing his genuine character, (NOT the one the media has forced down our throats through the years) while working several days on promos for Dick Clark's answer to "The View," a men's daytime talk show called "The Other Half," which ran for two years on NBC.

Danny is truly sincere and adores his family. Those of us Danny's age grew up with him. I watched him, humbled by years of personal demons, bad press and joblessness from which he had to start all over again, grateful for a second chance.

Back in the mid 1980s I was at a nightclub in the San Fernando Valley, where I grew up. I was shocked to see "Danny Partridge" working there as a DJ! It was surprising for me to see that, yet it showed he was willing to work and was not too proud, as some entertainers are. They are unable to evolve and are stuck in their past celebrity; they eventually disappear into obscurity.

Fast-forward to 2005. Danny was back in the spotlight, with a national TV talk show, radio show, and co-host of Dick Clark's daytime talk show, "The Other Half." He was the most appreciative of Dick Clark, who remembered his talent and likability. Danny realized he had been given another chance and wasn't about to screw it up. He was gracious, easygoing and, most important, humbled.

He was hilarious yet chivalrous. One day Dick Clark chastised me for taking my shoes off on the set. The female producer was concerned that my dark-bottomed shoes could mark up her white set as I stepped in to touch up Mario Lopez, Dick Clark and Danny. She gently requested that I remove my shoes. I did. A while later Dick Clark arrived on set. He barked "Young lady! What are you doing on a hot set with no shoes on? Do you know you could be electrocuted? Put those shoes back on right now!"

When Dick Clark is telling you off on a set, you want to run and hide, but Danny swooped in and saved me. I wasn't about to bust the producer, because I LIKE working in the business, but Danny did it for me. He jumped into the conversation, informed Dick that I was just doing what I was asked and didn't want to mark up the set, that I was just being a team player. It seemed to satisfy Dick Clark, and I was off the hook.

Danny said he knew he had to rescue me. And he did. Thank You, Danny.

Merv Griffin: Entrepreneur, Singer, Talk Show Host

People often ask me, of all the celebrities I have worked with, who is my favorite? It is most definitely Merv Griffin. He was a HUGE life-changer for me. You may know that Merv Griffin was one of the biggest success stories in Hollywood. He began his career as a crooner in a big band and became one of the wealthiest and most admired entrepreneurs in California. Creating game shows like "Wheel of Fortune" and being one of the longest-running talk show hosts are only a couple of his many business ventures. His immense success in real estate and hotel building is legendary.

We were shooting a magazine cover photo of Merv at his home, the Beverly Hilton Hotel. Merv arrived on set at the Hilton patio in a red shirt and was looking fit, healthy and happy. His silver hair, blue eyes and familiar smile disarmed me immediately.

He was in a jovial mood and made everyone around him feel comfortable. I went over to introduce myself and to begin his grooming for the shot. We instantly clicked. I don't know why, we just did.

Conversation flowed and he asked a lot of questions. Maybe that came from his years as a talk show host or maybe from all the wheeling and dealing he did. I've always observed in my career how the MOST successful people are easygoing and humble. He was the most real.

After several minutes of light conversation, as the crew buzzed around us setting up lights, props and discussing camera angles, Merv asked me if I would suggest what colors to wear for the shoot, although the wardrobe person had already chosen his attire. It was a sticky spot to be in, because you don't step on toes. However, it was Merv Griffin! So I agreed to come with him to choose.

That particular day the Vice President, Al Gore, was staying at the Beverly Hilton, on the wing where Merv had his expansive suite overlooking Santa Monica Boulevard.

Two men in black suits, just as in the movies, stood at the entrance to the elevator. Everyone was searched and the bags of those attempting to pass by the area were examined. Not everyone gets the chance to feel truly A-list, but I did that day, as Merv and I scooted by these guys, with no security check, even though I had my little black makeup box in hand.

Merv was a great conversationalist. We talked about some of the renovations going on at the hotel and his joy at the building of his long awaited dancing nightclub, the Coconut Grove, a dream of his. His idea of swing dancing coming back to its popularity of the 1940s was ahead of its time, because it took a while, but slowly it became all the rage again.

Merv obviously was ahead of his time in many areas. We entered his suite, a glamorous, grand apartment. His closet was immense. He had about ten shirts in different shades of blue, then there were the grey ones, red ones and white. It was a Disneyland of colored men's shirts.

How fun! He asked me to choose the best one that would bring out his eyes and skin color. I suspect this was all to make me feel special and important. I imagine being on TV all of those years, he had completely mastered what his best on-camera shade was, but it didn't matter to me then. He was in the moment with me, and I knew this afternoon with Merv Griffin would remain a lasting positive influence on me, which it most certainly has been.

I carefully studied all of the shirts in shades of blue and finally picked a sky-blue shade with a hint of gray. He smiled broadly, as if he was testing me and I passed. He changed from the red to the blue and we were off again, down the elevator and past the Secret Service guys, walking and talking, me and Merv.

We arrived on set to find everyone chilling, waiting on their special photo subject. The wardrobe girl slightly winced at the site of the newly chosen blue shirt, and I felt a tinge of guilt. I did explain to her that I wasn't a control freak and he had asked for my opinion. Although understanding my dilemma, she gently questioned me: How would I like it if the on-camera person asked her opinion on what color lipstick to wear? Got it. Lesson learned.

Now on to the life lesson of the day: Merv Griffin Listens. Sally makes her biggest career blunder!

In 1994, I was creating a bridal makeup kit and video. A bride could purchase a kit in one of three skin tones and have everything she needed to be gorgeous on her wedding day, her honeymoon and beyond. This product was ahead of its time, and I was excited!

While we were on set, the L.A. photographer Christopher Barr's assistant was inquiring about my new endeavor. "So tell me more about your bridal makeup kit. I might want to get that!" Merv was listening. A couple of minutes later he jumped in the conversation. "Ohhh. This sounds interesting! So the makeup kit is just for brides? And the video shows her how to use it? So, let me understand, these are not brides YOU are actually working on. How are these brides hearing about this product?"

Today when I watch "Shark Tank" and listen to the questions shot at these inventors, it brings me back to Merv Griffin and his questions of interest. I was a deer caught in the headlights. Everyone on set SHUT UP and waited to hear my response. It was like being caught with no underwear. Merv simply wanted to explore and gather more information, because that's what true entrepreneurs do.

I was mortified that I would be seen by anyone there or Merv Griffin himself as an opportunist. So what did I do? I feebly answered, giving some basic one-sentence responses, and quickly redirected the conversation back to anything ELSE we could talk about. Merv looked a bit puzzled for a moment and paused. His questions to me stopped. He turned to engage conversation with someone more interested in engaging with him.

Gone. I often think back to what coulda, shoulda, woulda happened with Merv and his obvious interest in my product. These missed opportunities in life that we experience are life altering. All I had to do was show my true excitement and authentic self about my product. I was more worried about what others may think. What had Dolly said? "Don't worry about what others think!"

Valuable lesson learned here. If someone is showing interest in you or your life, take ownership of it. Stand tall and talk about it. They wouldn't be asking you questions if they weren't interested.

If you make it up to the plate, don't be afraid to swing the bat!

Role Models

Paul Marciano: CEO

We named our beautiful, smart daughter Brigitte, after 1960s French actress Brigitte Bardot. She shares the blonde hair and brown eyes and, like Bardot, is strong of character and extremely photogenic.

It's clear to anyone who picks up a magazine or sees a billboard of a Guess clothing ad that brothers Paul and George Marciano designed the Guess campaigns with the image of Brigitte Bardot in their heads.

I was booked to work with Paul Marciano on a few occasions at his Los Angeles-based Guess headquarters.

On-location industrial-type shoots, in which the company is showcasing a CEO's ideas to his worldwide staff, are a great gig. I scoot in, prepare the talent for a quick shoot and I am done. I always learn something new and fabulous along the way.

After the introduction to this tall, silver- haired fashion merchandising genius and after being greeted in the French way with quick kisses on both cheeks, (I love that!) I immediately offered up the info that my daughter was named Brigitte. "How is it pronounced?" he inquired. I thought about that one for a second. "It's either Bri-git or Bri-jeet, depending whether the person pronouncing it is American or French." He agreed with a knowing smile, and from that moment, he was in the moment with me.

As the crew began setting up, he motioned to me. "Let's walk," he said, and I quickly caught up with his fast steps as we toured around the immense cement floored factory and he put out instructions to his staff along the way. As if I had paid for a guided tour, he carefully explained what was happening in each area, and I felt included. People like Paul Marciano are a quick judge of character, and if you pass the test, you are in and not forgotten.

The next time Paul Marciano and I met was about a year later. His first question?

"How is Bri-jeet?" Now that's a smart man. Can I say it again? I love my job.

Carson Daly: Television Host

Currently the host of "The Voice," Carson Daly doesn't do the celebrity vibe. He comes off as a laid back, regular guy, although he is very cute in person. During on camera grooming for public service announcements) for NBC's "The More You Know," he shared with me his resurgence into health and fitness, slimming down about 25 pounds. He took up cycling and changed his drink of choice from CC and Coke (that's my drink!) to white wine spritzers. When he started ordering this wussy cocktail, his friends would laugh and chortle when they went out on the town, but he stuck to those two healthy habits to change is physique forever. Thank you, Carson, for inspiring me. I listened.

Alicia Silverstone: Actress

My life lesson from Alicia is short, sweet and to the point. It happened on location in Westwood, doing makeup on Alicia Silverstone's promos for her TV show, "Miss Match." We broke for lunch, and Alicia took her dogs for a stroll. Yep. You guessed it. They pooped on the sidewalk. Alicia Silverstone, the star of the show, had her peeps right there with her, but she in no way expected or asked anyone to do her dirty work. She promptly scooped up the doggie poop and disposed of it. No star attitude from this very funny and beautiful comedienne and actress.

With all of the paparazzi activity surrounding celebrities, can we just get some stuff on film where celebs are being role models and doing some good things?

In Transition

Timothy Leary: Professor

"Turn on, tune in, drop out" were the words made internationally famous in the 1960s by Harvard Law professor and psychologist Timothy Leary. A genuine once-in-a-lifetime gig was being a fly on the wall (and makeup artist) for an interview series that explored Timothy Leary's final trip, dying. My job was to make him look a little healthier than he actually was. His death was near, as anyone who has seen a person in his or her last transition knows.

The glazed, lost eyes and sunken face startled me as I entered the makeup room to prepare him.

Soon I was to find that although his body was preparing to transition, he wasn't quite ready to go! His spunky, sarcastic delivery of one-liners and over-my-head transcendental ramblings of a man clearly caught up in his own infamy and belief systems made me take notice and pay attention. I didn't want to miss a thing. Clearly, this was going to be was one of those fasten-your-seatbelts experiences.

I think of him now in his made for TV royal blue jogging suit, which was meant to be worn by a man years younger and stronger but which somehow worked for him. In my two days with Timothy Leary, I bonded with him. How could you not? Like my mama, I've always been impressed and fascinated with education and life experience. This man, who may not have been popular, surely lived a life. He completely shared his strict and conservative upbringing, his early deadpan lifestyle and how simple experiences with drug experimentation led to a movement. His prison days allowed him encounters with an interesting selection of infamous people of his time, including Charles Manson. Manson sent him gifts that he refused. Manson desperately wanted to collaborate with him and repeatedly sent him grandiose ideas that fell on deaf ears.

A man ahead of his time, Leary was a man who happened upon a way to market himself that would land his name in the media, through one event that would label him forever in history. He was described by many accounts as a crazy case. I have decided that erudite types really hold a lot of power. It's what they choose to do with it that shapes their lives. Although he was conceited and omnipotent, there was a caring side too. He was concerned about our comfort, if we were bored, hungry or tired. Did we need to take a break?

On the second and last day, Mr. Leary seemed more tired, distant and a bit sad, too. We shot for only a couple of hours.

All the crew approached him one by one. They wanted pictures with this infamous man. The only one who didn't ask was me. (I have made it a practice to not ask for pictures with my clients). So Timothy Leary asked me if he could take his picture with me! It is a sweet, nice memory.

He passed away a short time later, his actual death, through his request, being recorded on video, and of course going viral on the Internet, with his last words: "Why Not?"

Bea Arthur: Actress

Comedy Central produced a series featuring comedians in their home environments, like a "Cribs" for the comedy world. I was booked to go to the home of "Golden Girls" and "Maude" fame, Bea Arthur, who was ill with cancer, and make her up for what promised to be a most insightful and amazing interview.

When I arrived at her Brentwood, Calif., home, two scary-looking Dobermans came charging full speed at my car door, barking and totally making eye contact. I'm like, "OK, I guess I'm not getting out of the car."

Seconds later, Bea Arthur appeared at the doorway. She got them to back off with a one word command: "Off!"

Her illness had wreaked havoc on her. She was emaciated and looked frail, but her fabulous Bea Arthur personality remained. I really wanted to make this woman look polished, and my talent was going to be put into full gear on this day. She was doing an on-camera interview, discussing her life in comedy, how storylines on TV changed over time, how they pushed the envelope and opened up discussions on topics like religion, homosexuality and racial bias. How the use of comedy in television helped to open people's minds: This was her specialty.

I told Bea Arthur that I knew and understood her understated look but that I was going to have to use lashes and more color and intensity to bring her out on camera. I was concerned what her response WOULD be, considering that this woman's famous strong presence was still very much alive, although her body was in decline. I will always remember her quick reply and enjoyed repeating it to my mom later that day: "Honey, you are gonna have to be a magician do something with this face. Whatever you gotta do. You gotta do your job and I gotta do mine." I said a little silent prayer and my hands went to work. I wanted so much to give this comedy icon the look that she deserved. Then the set was lit and the director called "action." The transformation of this entertainer was instantaneous!

Bea Arthur, as we all knew her, came to life, and the words flowed. Her eyes were sparkly bright as funny anecdotes continued throughout the process. I was appreciative that day of being part of it, and I always am, knowing that this was a moment in time that happens only once and that I was lucky to be there to experience it live and in person.

I have seen this process many times throughout my career from enduring celebrities who showed us all, with the steely focus, that the show must go on.

Bea Arthur passed away a few months later.

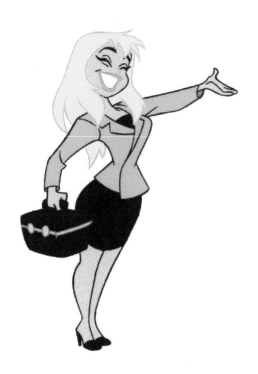

CHAPTER 6

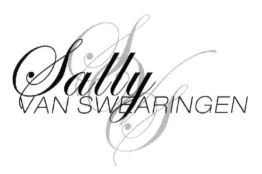

BEAUTY BEGINS THE MOMENT YOU DECIDE TO BE YOURSELF

COCO CHANEL

"Honey, Let Me Tell You..." Learn More From These Five Real Women

Intelligent, educated, real women have always inspired me. I decided to interview five inspirational ladies for this book, to get some insight from them about how they have reclaimed their own Beauty Power and what they really thought about the maturing process. It's wonderful to hear so much diversity on the subject. For example: On the topic of cosmetic surgery, would you or not? Some said "Go for it," Others said "I would never do it." Here's to real women and what truly makes them tick.

IT'S NOT OVER YET!

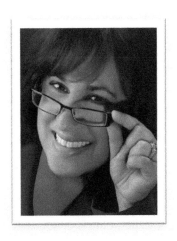

Judith Cassis, 54,

Hypnotherapist, Coach, Author

My best advice:
"Every life stage is beautiful."

What are your concerns about your looks and beauty power as you mature?

"I always had beautiful skin, but now in my 50s I have pigmented skin. I need to consider treatment for it, specifically. Beyond that, self-acceptance gives me peace."

What specific areas do you see are aging on your face, etc.?

"Smile lines."

What beauty tools, routines, products, exercises, mental mind-sets have you used that have kept you looking younger than your age?

"I stayed out of the sun, I use high quality skin care products, through the years I've had facials. I keep my face clean. I use relaxation techniques to deal with stress."

Are you in favor of cosmetic surgery, Botox, fillers, etc. to help reduce the look of aging?

"No. I believe in aging gracefully. Obsession with youth can hold us back from being what life intends for us as we mature. Every life stage is beautiful."

Have you done any of these?

"No."

What do you think of women who do not seem to accept the fact that they are maturing, who shop at teenagers' stores, dress in their daughters' jeans, wear Daisy Dukes and Ugg boots, etc.?

"We should dress the way we feel. If I looked good in Daisy Dukes, I would wear them! I don't."

At your place in life, what advice would you give to a woman who is entering the time you have already experienced?

"Accept yourself, make the most of what you have, focus on your inner beauty."

IT'S NOT OVER YET!

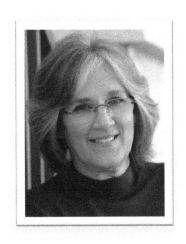

Circe Denyer, 62,

Author, Speaker, Technology Guru

My best advice:
"Eat well. Find out what your skin and inner self needs, as opposed to choosing general products that everyone uses."

What are your concerns about your looks and beauty power as you mature?

"I'm an entrepreneur, concerned that looks and age could affect getting a new client. Specifically, I wouldn't want to be seen as too old for the job."

What specific areas do you see are aging on your face, etc.?

"Dark circles under the eyes and where glasses are."

What beauty tools, routines, products, exercises, mental mind-sets have you used that have kept you looking younger than your age?

"I eat well and get plenty of sleep. I pay attention to my inner voice and emotions. Attitude affects our looks."

Are you in favor of cosmetic surgery, Botox, fillers, etc. to help reduce the look of aging?

"As an option others may make, I do not see this as a bad decision. I do see it as a personal choice.

Have you done any of these?

"No. I have not looked at my face or body and said, 'Oh, you need to change that.'"

What do you think of women who do not seem to accept the fact that they are maturing, who shop at teenagers' stores, dress in their daughters' jeans, wear Daisy Dukes and Ugg boots, etc.?

"I think those women don't have anyone telling them how beautiful they are. It is about acceptance and self-acceptance. It is one of my passions. I can tell you that there are beautiful women out there that believe they are not beautiful enough because they have no sense of acceptance or value from others or themselves."

At your place in life, what advice would you give to a woman who is entering the time you have already experienced?

"Eat well. Find out what your skin and inner self need, as opposed to choosing general products that everyone uses. Our skin is a reflection of what is going on inside. Make sure you are focused on inner wellness first."

IT'S NOT OVER YET!

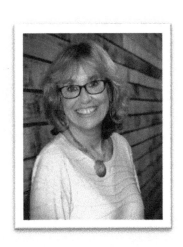

Linda Davies, 61,

Executive Director, Domestic Violence Center

My best advice:
"Who have I become?"

What are your concerns about your looks and beauty power as you mature?

"Those things aren't important to me. I'm not worried about looking too old. I don't get this thing when people say, 'You don't look your age!' What is that supposed to look like? If I'm going to be worried about that, why go out of the house?

"When I was younger I was told that I looked like Jane Fonda. That was nice. But I always felt that it was more my personality than my looks that made the impression. I was always able to chat my way through anything I wanted. **Beauty Power?** That has to come from within. I've had some really good Valentines Days. I don't have regrets."

What specific areas do you see are aging on your face, etc.?

"The lines around my mouth bother me, but the rest does not. It's just what our faces do. I smoked for years when I was younger, so they are most likely from that. My doctor tells me not to drink out of straws, and I don't. Other than that, I'm OK, really. If your face bothers you that much, put on some big sunglasses!"

What beauty tools, routines, products, exercises, mental mind-sets have you used that have kept you looking younger than your age?

"Skin care? Jojoba oil, because it's closest to your skin's natural oil, I have heard. I have a lot of energy, always have. I drink about 80 ounces of water every day and do a ton of walking, love to walk my dog. Four times a week I do some quick workouts with five-pound weights and elastic bands. I think staying active and having a sense of humor is key. I work with kids 50 to 60 hours a week. My friend went and spent $3,500 on a facial procedure. That was what she wanted to do for herself. I figured I should do something for myself too, so I spent $350 and had my teeth whitened."

Are you in favor of cosmetic surgery, Botox, fillers, etc. to help reduce the look of aging?

"If people want to, it's fine. I'd rather have people accept us as beautiful, aging women."

Have you done any of these?

"No. Not going to."

What do you think of women who do not seem to accept the fact that they are maturing, who shop at teenagers' stores, dress in their daughters' jeans, wear Daisy Dukes and Ugg boots, etc.?

"Instead of focusing on what you used to look like, maybe it should be how am I going to move into the next phase of my life?"

At your place in your life, what advice would you give to a woman who is entering the time you have already experienced?

"Before you go into menopause, go in and see a good doctor, figure out what vitamins you need to start on, be prepared before it happens. If you want to go ahead and go gray, do it before your body starts to look and feel it. I don't want to tell someone (a woman over 40) to stay out of the sun! Enjoy life! Kayak!

"What is the legacy you want to bring forward? Mine is I worked with young children and women who didn't have the resources to better themselves."

"Think about it this way: Who have I become?"

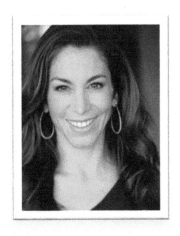

Melissa Rivera, 40,

Dancer and Actress

My best advice:
"Find what feeds your soul."

What are your concerns about your looks and beauty power as you mature?

"I'm not really concerned about losing **Beauty Power**, because at this point in my life I feel beautiful as I age. I do want to be healthy and radiant, and have great skin, like any woman would want. I think of my body as a temple and I take care of it.

"Here in L.A. and Hollywood, the importance of beauty and perfection is magnified, so of course there are some concerns, but I try not to obsess about it."

What specific areas do you see are aging on your face, etc.?

"Fine lines, droopy eyelids."

What beauty tools, routines, products, exercises, mental mind-sets have you used that have kept you looking younger than your age?

"I have a chemical peel every year, Obagi, since I was 34. I'm a dancer and work out and run every day one hour. I apply sunscreen several times a day. I always wear a long shirt, hat and sunglasses when I run. I protect my skin.

"I became a working dancer late in the game. I always wanted to be a dancer. Then I decided 'Why not?' And I went for it. I was 29 when I began, with ZERO experience. I started taking classes in popping and locking style. It takes a determination and discipline that is indescribable. It's an amazing process to be able to learn and then execute choreography on the highest level. To be able to dance alongside some of the best dancers in the world, it gives me an amazing feeling of confidence. Since dancing, I began to see a natural radiance that came from the inside; that nothing else has been able to do."

Are you in favor of cosmetic surgery, Botox, fillers, etc. to help reduce the look of aging?

"Yes, in moderation."

Have you done any of these?

"Botox."

What do you think of women who do not seem to accept the fact that they are maturing, who shop at teenagers' stores, dress in their daughters' jeans, wear Daisy Dukes and Ugg boots, etc.?

"Those women don't love themselves; really sad. Something inside that is obviously unfulfilled. They are searching for acceptance and confirmation of their beauty."

At your place in your life, what advice would you give to a woman who is entering the time you have already experienced?

"Try to RELAX. Accept the aging process with grace. I think about people who are born with life-debilitating illnesses and I am grateful that I can do what I do.

"The spiritual aspect of maturing is so important. You must feed your internal self, mind, soul and spirit.

"Dancing did that for me. It gave me an inner confidence. I have grown in certain places of my life because of dance. Find what feeds YOUR soul!"

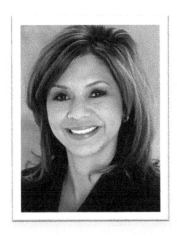

Dora Zavala, 50,

Mary Kay Beauty Director

My best advice:
"Just because they make it in your size
doesn't mean you should wear it."

What are your concerns about your looks and beauty power as you mature?

"Not so much physical appearance, like my face or overall look, more concerned about my weight/metabolism, body is changing. The physical changes that are occurring in my body as a result of maturing is what mentally impacts my **Beauty Power**."

What specific areas do you see you are on your face, etc.?

"Eyes. When I wake up I look in the mirror, more puffy, eyelids droop. My daughters, 26 and 21, say, 'Mom, you look tired.' It could have been cocktails, late evening. I'm passionate about my eyes, they are the windows of the soul. They tell if you are happy, sad, mad, but most importantly they tell your age."

What beauty tools, routines, products, exercises, mental mind-sets have you used that have kept you looking younger than your age?

"Routine. I use great, great products. I do a mask every Saturday morning. I get up and put on a revitalizing clay mask. Mary Kay Remask. I drink lots of water, been doing it for 20 years.

"We have a lot more women (our age) who have given up retaining their **Beauty Power** on purpose. WE do what WE do to retain our **Beauty Power**, to be a positive influence on other women.

I was running three-four times a week and kickboxing. Now I'm doing Zumba classes two-three times a week. Running was time to commune. I got so involved in the community that it took up space. Learning to create boundaries was what allowed me to get back to it. I created a zen room in my home and get on the treadmill at 4:30 a.m.

"I'm spiritual and have a strong faith. I have quiet time every morning. I read the Bible or some spiritual book. Sets my mind for the day. Also, journaling helps me reflect on the day, learn more about myself and helps me grow. Last year was a low spot. I sold my house, children moved out. I am alone for the first time in my life. I started to reflect: "Is this where I'm supposed to be in life?" I answered YES. This is exactly where I should be. I'm 50 and Fabulous!"

Are you in favor of cosmetic surgery, Botox, fillers, etc. to help reduce the look of aging?

"I'm not sure. I would try something on the eyelids."

Have you done any of these?

"No."

What do you think of women who do not seem to accept the fact that they are maturing, who shop at teenagers' stores, dress in their daughters' jeans, wear Daisy Dukes and Ugg boots, etc.?

"Just because they make it in your size doesn't mean you should wear it. These ladies have not learned to love themselves. Sad. I admire a woman who wears clothes that compliment her personal style. Dress for your audience. Am I going to a club or a business meeting?

A lot of **Beauty Power** comes from knowing who YOU are. I won't dress hoo-chee when I know I'm going to be in a room full of professional, respectable women. But later on I'll change into something fun and flirty."

At your place in your life, what advice would you give to a woman who is entering the time you have already experienced?

"See a doctor. Find out what is going in with your body. When I got hot flashes, immediately I did my research. Could it be my hormones? I take PMS vitamins.

Embrace who you are and the journey."

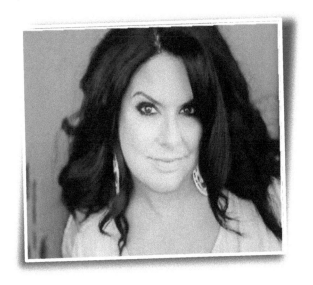

DeAnn Mitchell, 42,
Makeup and hair by Sally

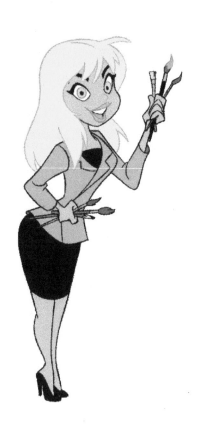

CHAPTER 7

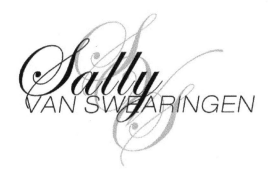

Sally
VAN SWEARINGEN

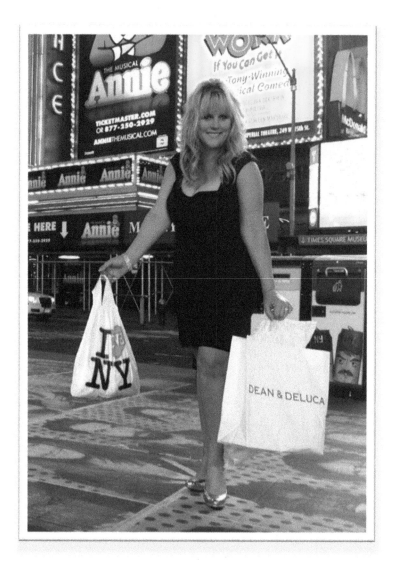

Having fun in Times Square.
It's Not Over Yet!

Self-Acceptance and Self-Love: Moving Forward

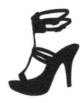

My Favorite Kind of People

My favorite kind of people are those who don't take themselves too seriously, are focused and live life. Usually my favorite people are some type of role model to me. People who JUST ARE.

They are getting stuff done. They are in the moment when they are with someone or doing a task. They look you in the eye when talking to you. They have nice things to say and notice when

217

something good is happening around them. Sometimes my favorite people just SHUT UP, so I admire that and try to be like them too (this one is challenging). My favorite people have goals.

Usually they accomplish them. And if they don't, they keep trying and give themselves credit for trying. My favorite people can make fun of themselves, too. They don't have to be the bitchin' one ALL the time. They let me be the bitchin' one too. I know when I am around my favorite people because they will always make me and others feel included. The most important thing I love about being around my favorite people is that they make me want to be a better person.

With this said, I'm going to open this final thought in "It's Not Over Yet!" by sharing an analogy from something learned from author and motivational speaker, Chellie Campbell.

Chellie makes looking at the relationships in our lives extremely simple. I like things simple. After learning her most basic and amusing analogy, the friendships and collaborations in my life changed, big time. I viewed people in an entirely new light. Thanks, Chellie. You so rock!!

Now, before I continue, you might wonder what do Chellie Campbell's analogies have to do with RECLAIMING OUR BEAUTY POWER.

Wait for it:

Chellie divides the world into two groups:

My People and Not My People

That's the gist of it, but here is more. In her book "Zero to Zillionaire," Chellie talks about the kind of people who ARE her people; they are Dolphins. NOT her people are Shark and Tuna. Get it so far?

Here are Chellie's words....

Dolphins

"Dolphins are friendly creatures, they swim in groups, they are intelligent and play and interact with each other. They have been known to ward off shark attacks and protect other fish in the sea. There are many accounts of Dolphins rescuing human beings.

People who are Dolphins are generous. They love to share the wealth. They'd like nothing better than everyone in the world to be rich, but they understand that you have to work for it. Because of this, they are wonderful mentors and teachers and are delighted to share their secrets of success with you. When you swim in the company of dolphins, you feel empowered, energized and uplifted. You feel better about yourself and the world around you, and you have more money too. Dolphins play win-win."

Now think of the people throughout your life who have helped elevate you or assisted you in any area of enrichment, without any expectation of personal gain, they just wanted to be helpful. These are the people we must most definitely stay with and search out. If they are in your life now, nurture the relationship. Next, open yourself up to meeting more like-minded people.

Let's explore WHO our Dolphins are; once we gather a list we see a commonality of the type of person we must be, and must be WITH, in our second half, to authentically reclaim our **Beauty Power,** and let's face it, just be happy.

I've compiled my list of Dolphins. There are hundreds of wonderful people who have assisted along the way, and you know who you are. The few names listed here tie in directly to the points I am making in this book. Thank you to these favorite people whom I have been blessed and fortunate to know and grow with:

Dr. Kenneth Davis, Michael Evans, Robin Becerra, Dr. Jill Strawbridge, John Mitchell, Carole Rosner, Michael Rooney, Emad Asfoury, Paddy Calistro, Harold Trenier, Bruce Leamon, Circe Denyer, Judith Cassis, Suzanne Bertsch, Arlyne Szerman, Jane Szerman, Lysa Nevarrez, Chris Clifford, Jeff Sterling, Jeannine Cascadden, David Glassman, Michael James, Sara Martin and Matt Randall.

WHO are YOUR Dolphins? Write them down. Acknowledge their help and guidance in your first half.

_____

_____

_____

_____

As we grow and move through this next chapter of our lives, we need more than ever to group with those people who understand and live this philosophy. This is the second half. Time to really LIVE it. For some of us, it can be the best and most fulfilling; for others it can be loneliness and despair, simply because we continue to hang with the same types of people who give us the same results.

This leads to the next of Chellie's groupings:

Sharks

"Sharks are eating machines. That is their sole purpose in life: eating. It's not their fault, they were born like that. They see everyone in the world as dinner. That includes you. Sharks are sometimes rich, but don't enjoy their wealth because the word "enough" doesn't exist in their vocabulary. Sharks don't share with anybody, because their constant thought is ME, me, me, I, I, I, so there is no room at the dinner table for anyone else except on a plate.

There are two kinds of sharks: angry sharks and con artist sharks."

Angry sharks

They are completely self-obsessed. They have no empathy for other people. You are food. They are angry with life and the world and are going to take it out on you. These sharks tend to scream and yell and throw tantrums in order to get their way. They will tell you everything that's wrong with YOU, if you give them an opportunity. Like if you say "Hello."

Con artist sharks

They are sharks in dolphin's clothing. (Sadly, this is an experience I put myself through way too many times!)

They pretend to be your friend and imitate dolphin behavior in order to get close to you. They have charisma and a ready smile, but look in their eyes; you'll see nothing but calculation.

They are running numbers, figuring what you are worth and how they can take advantage of you. Their offer sounds so fabulous! You suspect they are too good to be true, but what if it really is your lucky day at last and this is a fabulous opportunity for you to get rich?

Usually, the only ones getting rich are the sharks. They could pay you but why should they? They want all the goodies for themselves."

Thank you Chellie! At the end of the day, we like to socialize and drink wine with those people we love and admire, who make us feel good too. How often have you been in a group of otherwise awesome women and somehow a shark-like one is in the mix. How did this lady get in here? She over-compliments you while using condescending tones or expressions. When you are speaking, she is looking away, bored with you. You may not be doing business with her, but she is still a shark. She is not your friend and is not going to be. Let it go. It has nothing to do with you. Excuse yourself and move over to the dolphins, who love and respect you, and vice versa.

My friend Jill Strawbridge, whose doctorate is in human factors, sprang this on me in the 1990s and I never forgot it. She said, "You are at a cocktail party and someone comes over and presents a platter of shit. You can either accept it or say no thanks.

Say no thanks to the be-yatches. Something about being over 40, and especially over 50, gives us a power to behold. I just don't put up with nearly as much of that fake stuff as I did in my 30s, trying to get people to like me who just weren't going to anyway, even if I stood on my head. Instead, I gravitate to my dolphins.

Now the grouping no one wants to be categorized in:

Tuna

Tuna are the food for the sharks. They are the victims of the universe. They talk endlessly how awful life is and how badly they have been treated and how it isn't their fault. It's a one-way conversation, all they want from you is a sympathetic, "Oh poor thing!" now and then. Tuna complain a lot and don't accomplish much. They would love to share but they can't because they are broke."

I become uncomfortable when I am around a group of otherwise positive, exciting women, and a "Debbie downer" starts to complain, whine or gossip. I may make an attempt to change the subject, which sometimes works, because the power of dolphins in numbers is truly amazing to behold, but usually I just swim away as fast as possible.

Sometimes I find myself to be the one complaining or gossiping, but because of Chellie's teachings, combined with my own rediscovery of my **Beauty Power,** I find myself nipping it in the bud much faster than I did before.

WE are in our second half, and this time is for US!

Moving Forward

Recently two beautiful young hair stylists with loving spirits came to join my salon and taught me a few lessons. Our time with Samantha brought us a peaceful vibe and inspired us to keep the groove even more nurturing and professional. When Samantha walked in, we cleaned up our act. She set an example by simply living her life with high expectations of herself

Rae is a dynamo of talent and creativity, who continually brings learned and innate skills to our studio. Her energy and passion remind me of a 20-year old Sally just starting out. However, Rae figured out her style; edginess with a touch of class, way before I did.

I feel honored to be working with the next generation of beauty innovators, recognizing specific directions in them that they may not even have discovered themselves.

I love being a mentor to young talents entering the business. It is a responsibility that carries a lot of weight. I have to be accountable and authentic. I get a chance to do the things that I know could help move them to the next level. They teach me too, and we all help one another on our road to success. Dolphin Behavior

I have learned so many lessons, stepped over a lot of snakes and have survived stronger. Why would I NOT want to help a young person who is eager to grow and learn?

When you have the ability and power to help someone, why wouldn't YOU?

WHO can you guide and nurture, using your experience, expertise and life lessons?

Think of someone you can help and motivate. Write his/her name here:

_____

Contact him/her NOW! Offer your assistance.

I am willing to bet he or she will be blown away and will find life enriched by your act of kindness and generosity.

What's Next?

Are we going to travel? Mentor? Reward ourselves with fitness and health? Will we do a 5k, learn to tap dance, ride a Harley, hike Mount Everest and write a book?

I would be honored to hear from you, what you will accomplish and what you will gift yourself with.

Post 40, I had a baby, raised a daughter, went back to school to add an additional trade, created a makeup line, produced makeup videos, became a platform beauty educator, re-entered dance, created a new concept salon, wrote a book and mentored new artists along the way.

Post 50, there is more, a LOT more. Start now!

IT'S NOT OVER YET!

Make a list of five things you plan to do in the
next five years:

1. _____

2. _____

3. _____

4. _____

5. _____

What did you learn from "It's Not Over Yet!"?

_____

_____

_____

What have you learned about yourself?

_____

_____

_____

Are you reclaiming your **Beauty Power**? What steps have you taken to do this?

_____

_____

_____

What is the most important mind-set you will take with you from this book?

_____

_____

_____

_____

Thank you for coming along with me for the ride!

Truly enjoy and rock your **BEAUTY POWER!**

IT'S NOT OVER YET!

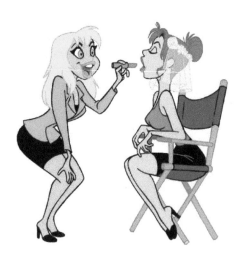

Sally's Favorite Products:

Studio Essentials Daily Moisture Protection,
broad spectrum SPF 15

Studio Essentials Amazing Tinted Primer

Studio Essentials BB cream

Studio Essentials Picture Perfect highlighting concealer

Studio Essentials Bronze Goddess all-in-one pencil

Studio Essentials Powderliner pencil

Ayur-Medic Enrichment cream

Ayur-Medic Retinol cream

To order go to: www.studio-essentials.com
Discount order code: **BPOWER**

Studio Essentials Cosmetics is
paraben-free, allergy tested
and always camera-ready.

"*I have used these fabulous products for
over 15 years to help maintain my Beauty
Power.*"

–Sally

My Products Order List:

_____

_____

_____

_____

_____

_____

_____

_____

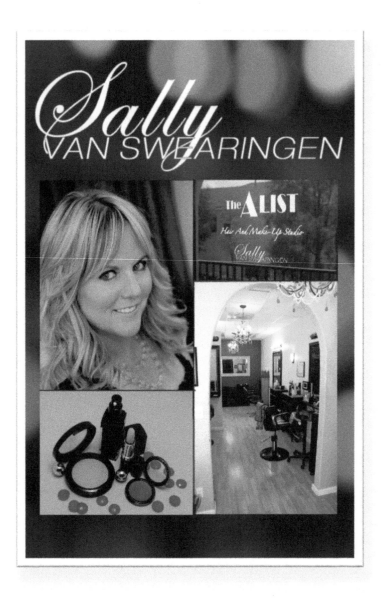

Sally Loves to Teach!

Sally is available for media, TV, radio, platform speaking and one-on-one consulting.

With her down to earth, humble yet funny style, Sally keeps her audiences smiling while they are getting gorgeous through simple, easy-to-follow examples and get-a-clue life experiences.

For more information on bringing Sally Van Swearingen to you or your event, email sally@itsnotoveryet.net.

Products may be purchased at:

www.Studio-Essentials.com

We want to hear your feedback!

How has "It's Not Over Yet!" shifted your thinking about YOUR BEAUTY POWER?

IT'S NOT OVER YET!

Please email your feedback to:

Sally@ItsNotOverYet.net

Sally Van Swearingen
MAKE-UP EXPERT!
www.SallyVanSwearingen.com

Author: It's Not Over Yet! - Reclaiming Your REAL
Beauty Power in your 40's, 50's and Beyond!
www.ItsNotOverYet.net

Creator: Studio Essentials Cosmetics:
www.Studio-Essentials.com

Salon: THE A-LIST Hair and Make-up Studio:
www.TheALISTscv.com

https://www.youtube.com/user/makeupedge

Salon: 661.260.1136

Credits

Production and Photography Director:

Matt Randall: Pro Photography Network

Photography:

Matt Randall: Pro Photography Network

Kirk McKoy: Twin Lens Photography (Cover Photography)

Emad Asfoury: LA Color Studio

Yoti Telio: Santa Clarita Photographic Studios

Jane Oncea: Fast Jayne Photography

Tara Rochelle: Tara Rochelle Photography

Nick Kosan: Nick Kosan Photography

Circe Denyer: Easybytes Training and Creative Technology

Robin Emtage: Robin Emtage Photography

Gary Choppe: Gary Choppe Advertising

Sarah Cascadden

Hair and Makeup for cover:

Patricia Norvell: Makeup

Rae Christman: Hair

IT'S NOT OVER YET!

Samantha DeNeal: Hair assist

Graphic Designers:

Sarah Cascadden

Dawn Teagarden: Teagarden Designs

Natasha David: (cover design)

Character Animation Designs:

Ken Boyer

Formatting:

Dawn Teagarden: Teagarden Designs

Circe Denyer: Easybytes Training and Creative Technology

Proofreading Services:

Tara Doherty

Kelsey Kilbury

Kathy Gosnell

Book Coach:

Judith Cassis: Success Made Simple

Notes

S A L L Y   V A N   S W E A R I N G E N

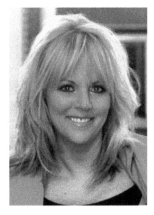 Is an internationally known, total beauty artist with a passion for bringing out a woman's best features to make her look and feel gorgeous.

Called "One of the Best Makeup Artists in the Country" by Allure Magazine, she has spent 26 years creating beauty as a makeup artist, esthetician and hair stylist.

She created a new niche in the 1990s as the Southern California bridal beauty guru. Her Bridal Makeup Studio transformed over 3,000 brides.

Sally next set her sights on showing others how to get gorgeous through her Los Angeles-based TV show Makeup Trends, and her educational makeup technique courses for makeup artists, revealing simple beauty tricks that transform a woman in minutes. Celebrities, CEOs, brides, Olympic athletes and real women of all shapes and sizes have been inspired by Sally Van Swearingen's beauty wisdom.

Sally and her team create flawless makeup and hair looks in her salon, The A LIST Hair and MakeUp Studio in Santa Clarita, Calif. She continues to blog on all things beauty and will be a working makeup and hair artist until she can't hold a brush. With a fresh start post 50, Sally has one amazing daughter, two dogs and a kitten. She plans to be a beautiful bride in her second half.

Author's Note - January, 2015

I am beyond thrilled how well this book is being received by women! But, why should I be surprised?

Our time has come, and it is now.

For me it started when I read a story about Sharon Stone in People magazine how she rocks her look post 50. Then several features celebrating actresses pushing the beauty envelope post 40, grabbing roles of maturing beauties, instead of times past where, at a certain age they were relegated to plain Jane mom or grandma status. Christie Brinkley in a bathing suit at 60 looking like her authentic self was a breath of fresh air. Even our latest 'Bond' woman, actress Monica Bellucci, to be featured in the next James Bond film is 50!

The internet site Huff/Post 50 gives us a daily Disneyland of opportunities, showcasing amazing, accomplished, gorgeous women.

It's definitely NOT over yet!

Sally Van Swearingen

CPSIA information can be obtained
at www.ICGtesting.com
Printed in the USA
JSHW021404051219
2806JS00003B/5

9 780990 304760